THE CURIOUS WORLD
OF DRUGS AND THEIR FRIENDS

INGO NIERMANN is a writer living in Berlin. Working both in fiction and nonfiction, he is a contributor to a number of international magazines such as *032c*, *Abitare*, *Kid's Wear*, and German *Vanity Fair*. He is the inventor of "The Great Pyramid," a project under development that seeks to erect a common memorial and gravesite on a massive scale, and recently published *Solution 9: The Great Pyramid*.

ADRIANO SACK is a writer living in New York. He is working for various German publications such as *Architectural Digest*, the art magazine *Monopol*, and *Liebling*. He recently launched the fashion website ilikemystyle.net. His next book, *Gebrauchsanweisung für die USA* (*Users Guide to the USA*), a witty analysis of contemporary America, is due to be published in Germany in fall 2008.

THE CURIOUS WORLD OF DRUGS AND THEIR FRIENDS

A Very Trippy Miscellany

INGO NIERMANN AND ADRIANO SACK

TRANSLATION BY AMY PATTON

A PLUME BOOK

PLUME
Published by the Penguin Group
Penguin Group (USA) Inc., 375 Hudson Street, New York, New York 10014, U.S.A.
Penguin Group (Canada), 90 Eglinton Avenue East, Suite 700, Toronto, Ontario, Canada M4P 2Y3 (a division of Pearson Penguin Canada Inc.)
Penguin Books Ltd., 80 Strand, London WC2R 0RL, England
Penguin Ireland, 25 St. Stephen's Green, Dublin 2, Ireland (a division of Penguin Books Ltd.)
Penguin Group (Australia), 250 Camberwell Road, Camberwell, Victoria 3124, Australia
(a division of Pearson Australia Group Pty. Ltd.)
Penguin Books India Pvt. Ltd., 11 Community Centre, Panchsheel Park, New Delhi – 110 017, India
Penguin Group (NZ), 67 Apollo Drive, Rosedale, North Shore 0632, New Zealand
(a division of Pearson New Zealand Ltd.)
Penguin Books (South Africa) (Pty.) Ltd., 24 Sturdee Avenue, Rosebank, Johannesburg 2196,
South Africa

Penguin Books Ltd., Registered Offices: 80 Strand, London WC2R 0RL, England

Published by Plume, a member of Penguin Group (USA) Inc. Originally published under the title *Breites Wissen: Die seltsame Welt der Drogen und ihrer Nutzer* in Germany.

First American Printing, September 2008
10 9 8 7 6 5 4 3 2 1

Translation copyright © Ingo Niermann and Adriano Sack, 2008
All rights reserved

Illustrations by Shingo Kuchiki and Brook Banham/Middlecott

Ⓟ REGISTERED TRADEMARK—MARCA REGISTRADA

LIBRARY OF CONGRESS CATALOGING-IN-PUBLICATION DATA

Niermann, Ingo, 1969-
    [Breites Wissen. English]
    The curious world of drugs and their friends : a very trippy miscellany / Ingo Niermann and Adriano Sack.
        p. cm.
    "A Plume book."
    Originally published under title : Breites Wissen : die seltsame Welt der Drogen und ihrer Nutzer."
    ISBN 978-0-452-28991-8
    1. Drug abuse—Miscellanea. 2. Psychotropic drugs—Miscellanea. 3. Celebrities—Drug abuse—Miscellanea. I.
Sack, Adriano. II. Title.
    HV5801.N554 2008
    362.29—dc22

                                                                                    2008017068
Printed in the United States of America
Designed by Judith Banham/Middlecott

THE CURIOUS WORLD
OF DRUGS
AND THEIR FRIENDS

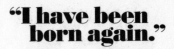

"I have been born again."

Cary Grant, *about his year*
of weekly LSD trips

ANIMALS ON

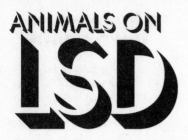

CATS lose their fear of dogs, bat the air, and salivate. They toy with mice instead of eating them. One mother cat allowed a mouse to suckle her.

MICE pack their bodies into a furry ball in a corner of their cage to avoid contact with sober conspecifics. When alone, they gnaw any object placed in front of them or in general behave inexplicably.

SPIDERS given low doses weave their webs with exceptional regularity, achieving greater perfection than ever before. At higher doses they spin only loose, disconnected threads.

HORNETS AND WASPS become oversensitive and show aggression toward their colony.

FISH appear confused, stop having sex, and cease to care for their young. The school disperses.

PIGEONS isolate themselves from sober fellows and form a subgroup. They ignore mating signals and nest duty and stop caring for their feathers.

RATS show poor orientation during maze experiments and run into walls just as often as blind rodents do.

GOATS walk in geometric paths, forming squares, figure eights, or Ls.

TOADS AND NEWTS are drained of skin color.

Cutting Agents

FOR HASHISH OR SUBSTANCES FRAUDULENTLY SOLD AS HASHISH

The cutting agents are kneaded into the hash by hand if the consistency allows. Otherwise, hash bricks are placed upon a hard, flat surface (usually in the purchasing dealer's country), covered with the cutting agent, and ironed in with an electric iron.

★ henna powder ★ tree resin ★ vegetable oil ★ ash ★ candle wax ★ tar
★ turpentine ★ powdered milk ★ mulberry juice ★ condensed milk
★ pomegranate juice ★ butter ★ fruit paste ★ shoe polish ★ mosquito spirals
★ dung (especially camel dung) ★ car tires ★ kneaded cake dough
★ play dough (as the especially soft "black Afghan") ★ sand ★ dust ★ soup cubes

PLACES

MADE FAMOUS BY DRUGS

☆ CHRISTIANIA/COPENHAGEN

Hippies and squatters took over a group of abandoned military barracks here. After several failed attempts to clear the area, the city of Copenhagen tolerates the community as a self-governing district. Christiania calls itself "Freetown Christiania," flies its own flag, and allows cannabis to be both openly sold and consumed on the premises. A raid of "Pusher Street" in 2003 did, however, result in the arrest of more than fifty dealers. The future of Christiania remains uncertain.

☆ TIJUANA/MEXICO

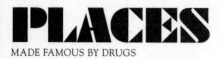

The most popular Mexican border town is only a quick trip from San Diego; just park in a border parking lot and walk over. Here you'll find not only alcohol, but prescriptions and any other kind of drug imaginable, along with prostitutes of all ages, shapes, and genders. No ID required.

☆ LAS BARRANQUILLAS/MADRID

This Madrid shantytown counts as Europe's leading cocaine and heroin shipping hub; stilted homes selling drugs out of barred drive-thru-style windows are nearly impregnable to police. A fire is kept burning at every sales station. As soon as the police snitch sounds the alarm, all of the goods are tossed into the fireplace and burned. In the early days, a police officer would shimmy onto the roof and pour water down the chimney to save the evidence, so residents built twenty-foot chimneys. Nearly a half million syringes were seized in the settlement in 2004 alone. Las Barranquillas's days are numbered; a new highway and railway are scheduled to be built on the site. The drug clans have already set up operations in another part of town, El Salobral.

☆ BAHNHOF ZOO/BERLIN

West Berlin's former main train station (downgraded to a regional train station in 2006) and without a doubt one of the shabbiest transportation centers in preunified Germany. The memoirs of the heroin-addicted "Christiane F." made its name a synonym for druggie land.

☆ NORMAN'S CAY/BAHAMAS

Little island in the Bahamas, forty-five miles southeast of Nassau. Big-time dealer Carlos Enrique Lehder Rivas nested here in 1977, built his own airstrip, and turned the entire island into a cocaine trafficking headquarters. Having driven all of the other island residents away, he threw raucous, heavily-armed parties, of which nothing remains today except for a rusty airplane wreck just off the island.

☆ WOODSTOCK/NEW YORK

A massive open-air concert took place here in 1969, on a farmer's alfalfa field in Bethel, New York, forty miles outside of Woodstock. Often considered the high point of the hippie movement, legendary drug friends such as Jimi Hendrix, Sly and the Family Stone, Joe Cocker, and Crosby, Stills, Nash and Young all gave performances. The weather was bad, but everyone shared their LSD. Two people died during the four-day festival—one from a heroin overdose, and the other was run over by a tractor.

☆ GOA/INDIA

Meeting Maharishi Mahesh Yogi in 1967, the Beatles proved themselves just as good at freeloading as they did when they stole Ken Kesey's idea for the *Magical Mystery Tour*. India was all the rage in Western counterculture circles. In the Indian state of Goa, located on the country's western coast, dropouts and longtime vacationers gathered to smoke pot, drop acid, try opium, and air out their naked bodies. A new kind of colonialism was born: native culture corruption via sympathy-soaked loitering. True Goans took the country route ("Hippie Trail") on into Turkey, Iran, Afghanistan, and Pakistan, then stayed a while for the cheap dope in Istanbul or Kabul before scrounging another ride with the next wave of hippies. Goan subculture flowered most recently with techno trance enthusiasts in the early nineties.

☆ ZABRISKIE POINT/CALIFORNIA

Zabriskie Point is a section of California's Death Valley. The legendary sociologist Michel Foucault took LSD here in 1967 (and then again in the gay saunas of New York), and Michelangelo Antonioni shot a scene here for his 1970 film of the same name, known for its deeply meaningful trippiness: First there is only one single naked couple, then suddenly hundreds rolling around, making love on the gravelly side of a boulder. The consciousness-expanding, dramatic, and surreal expanses of the Zabriskie Point landscape were formed 5 million years ago when a lake evaporated; it is named after the manager of a railroad company.

☆ CHELSEA HOTEL/NEW YORK

"*Here's room 115, filled with S&M queens,*" Nico sang in "Chelsea Girl"—one of the countless songs about the 23rd Street hotel. Artists, poets, and musicians lived here (Frida Kahlo, Jean-Paul Sartre, Leonard Cohen); this is where Warhol shot a movie and the heroin-addicted Sex Pistol Sid Vicious stabbed his girlfriend Nancy Spungen. Presumably there is no drug that has not been massively consumed in these rooms. In 1993, gallery owner Gavin Brown was the first to exhibit the work of the painter Elizabeth Peyton in room 828.

FRIEND NUMBER 1
Boy George

"Heroin was maybe the worst drug I took. But I didn't realize that until I didn't have any left," explained the pop star, who, at the height of his addiction, introduced himself as *"your favorite junkie"* at a 1986 benefit concert protesting South African apartheid. That same month, keyboard player Michael Rudetski died of an overdose in Boy George's apartment.

Boy George was born George Alan O'Dowd in 1961 in the southern English town of Eltham. As the heavily made-up and outlandishly costumed lead singer of the band Culture Club, he became an androgynous world star with his 1982 hit "Do You Really Want to Hurt Me?"

"I would rather have a cup of tea than sex," he once said when asked about his sexual orientation. But Boy George, who was at the time involved in a turbulent relationship with his drummer, Jon Moss, soon gravitated toward harder drugs. In 1986, as his band was already in the process of breaking up, the British tabloid *Sun* ran a cover story with the headline "Boy George Has Only Eight Weeks Left to Live." After a stint in rehab, the singer founded the House project Ezzee Possee ("Everything starts with an E") and later appeared with the band Jesus Loves You as Angela Dust. In 2003 Boy George, who by then was working mainly as a DJ, moved to New York for *Taboo*, the Broadway musical starring himself in the role of performance artist Leigh Bowery. The show closed after a less than three-month run.

On October 7, 2005, the entertainer made a 3 a.m. emergency call to police reporting a burglary in his Little Italy apartment. But officers arriving on the scene found no intruder, only a shaken Boy George and *"about five grams of a banned substance"* on his computer desk. The substance, to be precise, was an eighth of an ounce of cocaine in thirteen small plastic bags. In June 2006, Boy George was sentenced to five days of community service cleaning the streets of New York.

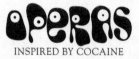

OPERAS

INSPIRED BY COCAINE

◎ HÉRODIADE (1881) by Jules Massenet ◎ THAÏS (1894) by Jules Massenet ◎
◎ SALOME (1905) by Richard Strauss ◎ ELECTRA (1907) by Richard Strauss ◎
◎ MOSES AND ARON (1925) by Arnold Schoenberg ◎
◎ WOZZECK (1925) by Alban Berg ◎ OEDIPUS REX (1927) by Igor Stravinsky ◎
◎ ARABELLA (1932) by Richard Strauss ◎

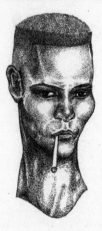

FRIEND NUMBER 2
Grace Jones

Given the local habit, it may seem like a difficult thing to be charged with drug possession in Jamaica, but Grace Jones (born 1948) managed. The model-turned-pop-star-re-mained-model has been partying since the seventies and has always had a knack for tumultuous situations: She once aimed a water gun at Andy Warhol, causing him to lose his platinum-blond wig (much to his embarrassment) and smacked a British talk-show host who dared to turn his back to her to speak with another guest. During a fashion show performance for British hat designer Philip Treacy, she fell from her chair (but kept singing while lying on the floor). Jones, whose photo in an Armani jacket was the definition of gender-bending coolness for a decade, has not produced any significant record since her 1987 concept album, *Slave to the Rhythm*. "We're nightclubbing. Bright-white clubbing. Oh isn't it wild," she sang in her cover version of a David Bowie/Iggy Pop song. She stuck to the concept and still makes the notoriously excessive Naomi Campbell look like a mild-mannered saint.

WHAT
COCAINE DOES:

GOTTFRIED BENN—"O NIGHT" (1916)

O Night! I've already taken cocaine,
and blood dispersion's underway,
Hair turns grey, the years race by,
I must, I must in ardour
Bloom just one more, before it's over.
O Night! I ask so little.
A tiny piece accumulation,
An evening fog, a congestation
of space collapse, of self-perception. (. . .)
O Hush! I sense a tiny ramming:
It stares at me—it is no taunt—:
Face, I: me, lonely God,
Converging grandly 'round a thunderbolt.

EXCEPTIONAL METHODS

FOR CONSUMING CANNABIS

THE BURROW

☮ This technique is considered a must for nature lovers, who can appreciate both the smoke's earthy smell and the intensive nature experience felt while stoned in these surroundings. A branch is used to dig two holes, forming a V-shaped tunnel in the ground. The chillum, a small sieve in which the marijuana or tobacco-hashish mixture is lighted, is inserted into one end of the passageway while the smoker inhales the earth-cooled, lightly seasoned smoke from the other. Another possibility includes digging a somewhat larger hole and inserting a bottomless bottle (*1*). You place the piece containing the smoke product in the bottle top and draw from the other side of the burrow, preferably using the proper setup (*2*), but purists suck the smoke directly from the ground (*3*).

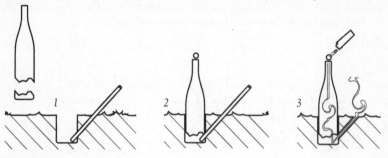

THE SOUTHERN CROSS

☮ Four holes, one pointing in each cardinal direction, are punched in a cardboard toilet paper core or, better yet, the longer cardboard core from a paper towel roll. Now all that's left to do is roll the joints; each joint is inserted into one of the holes and sealed around the edges with candle wax. Smoke is drawn from one end of the cardboard tube after all of the joints have been lit at once, though the opposite end must be held closed with a hand.

THE VAPORIZER

☮ In a vaporizer (inhaler), weed or hashish is heated only until the active ingredient begins to evaporate. This prevents inhaling other by-products such as tar or carbon monoxide. Vaporizers can be purchased in medical specialty shops or head shops and are especially helpful to nonsmokers wishing to ease THC inhalation.

THE DEATH STAR

✌ A construction made of eight, ten, or twelve empty bottles arranged in a circle. A hole is drilled in the middle of each bottle, and each is fitted with a chillum containing the marijuana or hashish-tobacco mixture. A hose system pulls the smoke across one or two water containers, enabling the smoker to inhale from all eight, ten, or twelve mixtures at once. Instructions abound on the Internet—Death Star assembly requires a foundation course in measurement and control technology.

THE BUCKET

✌ Fill a bucket with water, then find a large plastic soda bottle and cut off the bottom. Unscrew the top, cover the bottle top with aluminum foil, and place the construction in the bucket (*1*). The bottle should be submerged, with only the mouth of the bottle protruding out of the water. Perforate the aluminum foil with a ballpoint pen or pencil, place the dope or grass on top, and light it (*2*), pulling the bottle very slowly upward (*3*). Pressure should pull the smoke downward, into the bottle. When the bottle is almost completely out of the water (do not pull it all the way out!), remove the foil, put your lips over the hole, and inhale, pushing the bottle slowly back into the water. This surefire method quickly draws 1 to 1.5 liters of smoke into the lungs.

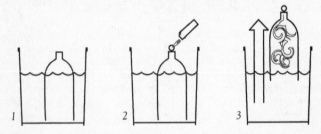

THE APPLE

✌ Bore a hole in an apple. The user then secures the joint or chillum to one end and inhales the smoke from the other. A slightly more refined version: Drill another hole perpendicular to the previous one. The chillum is secured to the top and the user holds the second hole closed while inhaling. Then, when the aromatic, intoxicating smoke enters the lungs, the third hole is opened to "drag" a last bit of air through to the end. This is as refreshing and flavorful as the burrow, though completely different in terms of taste.

PEACH SCHNAPPS PIPE

✌ Fill a water pipe with peach schnapps. The smoke takes on a pleasant, fruity smell, and the alcohol somehow intensifies the drug effect. Braver smokers might also try drinking the schnapps afterward.

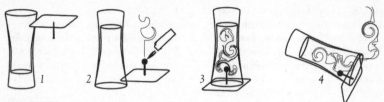

THE GLASS

✌ Poke a sewing needle through a beer coaster (*1*). Affix a clump of hash to the tip of the needle and light (*2*). Now put a glass upside-down over the hashish (*3*). As soon as the glass is filled with smoke, the user puts his lips to the edge, quickly lifts the coaster, and sucks the entire "hit" from the glass (*4*). Wait until the glass fills up with smoke again and pass to the next person.

HOW 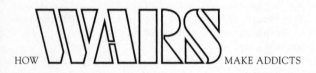 MAKE ADDICTS

THE CRUSADES (STARTED IN 1096)
In Europe, opium had all but disappeared when Christianity began to spread. It took the Christian crusades in the Orient to bring it back again.

THIRTY YEARS' WAR (1618–1648)
Helped to spread tobacco use in Europe.

OPIUM WARS (1840–1843 AND 1856–1860)
According to author Chalmers Johnson, the British Empire *"operated the world's largest and most successful drug cartel."* The wars against China were intended to force the country to import opium from India, a stronghold of British imperialism at the time. Opium was declared illegal in 1729, but the British East India Company needed money to finance its operations in South and Southeast Asia. Approximately nine hundred tons of opium were smuggled into China via Bengal in the 1820s. In a letter to Queen Victoria in 1839, the Confucianist commissioner Lin Zexu wrote: *"I give you my assurance that we mean to cut this harmful drug forever."* Two wars later, in 1860, the Chinese signed the Treaty of Tianjin, effectively legalizing opium import. The Australian scholar Carl A. Trocki maintains that *"without the drug, there probably would have been no British Empire."*

AMERICAN CIVIL WAR (1861–1865)
AND THE FRANCO-GERMAN WAR (1870–1871)
Morphine injections were introduced as a pain reliever for injured soldiers.

WORLD WAR I (1914–1918)
The London department store Harrods sold packets containing morphine,

cocaine, a needle, and a syringe under the slogan "A Useful Present for Friends at the Front." Many injected war invalids later became addicts, among them high-ranking Nazi official Hermann Göring.

WORLD WAR II (1939–1945)
The airborne soldiers in particular were no strangers to stimulants. The Germans issued Pervitin (methamphetamine) and Scho-ka-kola (highly caffeinated chocolate). In 1944, the German Wehrmacht developed a "miracle drug" under the project code name D-IX. The substance was a mixture of cocaine, Pervitin, and the opiate Eukodol. Concentration camp prisoners given the drug were forced to shoulder a fifty-pound assault pack and walk around in a circle until they collapsed in exhaustion.

KOREAN WAR (1950–1953)
American GIs were partial to amphetamine (speed) injections—especially when mixed with heroin.

SUEZ CRISIS (1956)
After being voted out of office, Sir Anthony Eden, British prime minister from 1955–1957, confessed that he had been high on speed during the entire Suez Canal conflict.

VIETNAM WAR (1962–1973)
Approximately 200 million amphetamine doses were distributed among U.S. troops. Many soldiers became heroin addicts. Drug abuse accounted for more casualties than war injuries did.

SOVIET-AFGHAN WAR (1979–1989)
Many Soviet soldiers returned home as junkies and stoners.

U.S. WAR ON IRAQ AND AFGHANISTAN (SINCE 2001)
Returning U.S. soldiers suffering from recurrent nightmares and post-combat trauma were given ecstasy in an experimental trial in South Carolina. Ecstasy apparently helps the soldiers "open up" and speak freely about their experiences.

COUNTRIES IN WHICH DRUG DISTRIBUTION AND POSSESSION IS PUNISHABLE BY **DEATH**

🗡 Algeria 🗡 Bahrain 🗡 China 🗡
🗡 Cuba 🗡 Egypt 🗡 Gambia 🗡 India 🗡
🗡 Indonesia 🗡 Iran 🗡 Laos 🗡 Malaysia 🗡
🗡 Mali 🗡 Myanmar 🗡 Oman 🗡
🗡 Pakistan 🗡 Philippines 🗡 Qatar 🗡
🗡 Singapore 🗡 South Korea 🗡 Sri Lanka 🗡
🗡 Syria 🗡 Taiwan 🗡 Thailand 🗡
🗡 United Arab Emirates 🗡 Vietnam 🗡 Yemen 🗡

Helmut Berger's DRUG SHEET

The Austrian actor has a well-known penchant for excess. He was Luchino Visconti's long-time lover and worked with the Italian film legend on *The Damned* and *Conversation Piece*, among others. Berger lost his grip after the director's death but made a kind of comeback in the eighties as Fallon Carrington's roguish lover in the TV series *Dynasty*. In his autobiography, *Ich*, Helmut Berger (born 1944) gives a flowery account of his experiences with various drugs. Especially striking: At the Red Cross Ball in Monaco, after doing a powerful line of cocaine, he came back to his table and defecated in his white tuxedo pants. In an effort to conceal the faux pas, Berger remained seated throughout the evening (snubbing the female companions at the table who wanted to dance) and complained loudly of the offensive smell wafting off of the Monaco harbor and into the ballroom.

✻ ✻ ✻

HASHISH After coming to London in the 1960s, Berger befriended photographer David Bailey, Cat Stevens, and Mick Jagger. Journalists eager to report on the new Flower Power Generation brought *"the hash straight to our house, so that we could feed them stories."* He went to a party hosted by Jack Nicholson while working on the *Dynasty* set in the eighties: *"We smoked a few joints and horsed around a little."* The excursion nearly cost him his contract when producers found out.

✻ ✻ ✻

LSD In 1970, the producer of the musical *Hair* gave Berger a *"four-cornered, finger-thick brown chunk, like a raisin,"* his first trip. *"And the leaves really were breathing my breath, the branches of the tree enfolded me gently."* His childhood sweetheart Yla Suchanek, a longtime lover of the Persian Shah, appeared to him like *"one of those healthy cows in the Alps, like the smiling lavender cow on Milka bar wrappers."*

✻ ✻ ✻

OPIUM Opium, like cocaine, was among Berger's "happymakers." He smoked it for the first time in 1974 at a horse race in the desert, *"Unlike LSD, you don't see any astonishing pictures, it just relaxes you in a way that not even the best sex can."* Berger lay in a Bedouin tent the entire evening and made *"relaxed conversation in all languages."*

✻ ✻ ✻

ECSTASY Berger took his first hit of ecstasy in Paris in 1985 and washed it down with wine. He was overwhelmed by an *"immense urge to cuddle, but without necessarily wanting to attack."* He found having sex in this condition fairly ordinary, but he did, however, enjoy six to eight orgasms in his mind. Berger warns against combining ecstasy with alcohol, since it causes the head to *"shatter in 1,000 pieces."*

COCAINE In 1971, when Berger took the *"absolute jet set drug"* at the Number One nightclub in Rome: *"I wanted to be 'in.' Back then. Soon I was tossing back half a kilo."* Later he bought a solid gold drinking straw, custom made by Bulgari. For Berger, this particular high exceeded all other drugs. *"I can work, dance, jerk around for two, three days in a row."* When the effects wear off, the *"sex was just totally unbridled."*

He served *"cocaine by the soupspoon"* at his forty-eighth birthday party. Today, Berger demonstrates *"against hard drugs at anti-drug conventions."*

✳ ✳ ✳

ALCOHOL Even his alcohol-bingeing days are behind him, after good friends had run away in droves. Berger's drinking became increasingly heavy after the death of his lover Luchino Visconti in 1976, and he became, as German television audiences know, *"the opposite of what I really am. A person that I hate with every fiber of my being."*

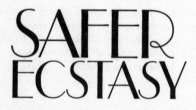

SAFER ECSTASY

Taking ecstasy leads to an increased production of free radicals, and repeated use can damage serotonin receptors (important for a sense of well-being) and cause memory disturbance. To prevent this, the British drug utopist David Pearce (author of *The Hedonist Imperative*) recommends the following counteragents:

✳ VITAMIN C
✳ VITAMIN E
✳ ZINC
✳ ASPIRIN
✳ SSRI ANTIDEPRESSANTS SUCH AS PROZAC OR ZOLOFT. (Only after the high. Using both at the same time will weaken the ecstasy's effect. But taken afterward, they restore sunken serotonin levels and brighten the mood.)

TO PREVENT DEHYDRATION AND OVERHEATING: Drink lots of water, but no more than a half-liter per hour. Consuming too much water and too little salt causes the internal organs to swell, and increased pressure on the brain stem can lead to coma and death. Isotonic beverages such as Gatorade are ideal— but avoid drinking alcohol, which only increases the risk of overheating and dehydration. Alcohol plays a role in most ecstasy-related deaths.

FOR IMPURITIES: If you're lucky, the MDMA has only been cut with starch or talcum powder. Usually MDMA is combined with other stimulants such as speed, caffeine, and ephedrine or with hallucinogenic substances such as 2C-B or LSD. Rare ecstasy pills have also been found with DXM—a cough suppressant with psychedelic properties—and PXM, a highly toxic hallucinogen. Those who prefer to play it safe can order ecstasy testing kits online—discrete packaging is guaranteed.

FRIEND NUMBER 3
Yves Saint Laurent

"He was born with a nervous breakdown," his one-time-lover
and business partner (and bodyguard and doormat and press
agent) Pierre Bergé said about him. Arguably the most important fashion designer of the twentieth century, Saint Laurent
was born in 1936 in the Algerian harbor city of Oran. He became the successor to Christian Dior at age twenty-one, but
was drafted into the military three years later. Sensitive Saint
Laurent was mentally unable to cope with the soldier's life and
was transported to the Parisian military hospital Val-de-Grâce,
where he was treated with electroshock therapy and tranquilizers.

Directing his own label from triumph to triumph in the years
after, Saint Laurent battled his anxieties with sedatives and gin and experimented with practically every other substance as well. The excesses in his Moroccan
villa are legendary; one member of his entourage even managed to shock Mick Jagger
by offering him heroin at a wedding. When Saint Laurent's longtime muse Loulou de
la Falaise showed him how to chew hashish instead of smoking it, he was flabbergasted:
"Well, that day he had eaten the whole thing." His love affair with Jacques de Bascher in
1973 seems to have been a turning point. Previously his drug of choice had been marijuana; Bascher drew him into more excessive circles, both sexually and with drugs.

One of his most successful perfumes goes by the name of Opium. In the early nineties, he was lethargic from tranquilizers and bloated from twenty-five Coca-Colas a day.
In his retirement letter from the fashion house he founded, Saint Laurent wrote: *"I have
known fears and the terror of solitude. I have known those fair-weather friends we call
tranquilizers and drugs. I have known the prison of depression and the confinement of
hospital. But one day, I was able to come through all of that, dazzled yet sober."* In June
2008 he died of brain cancer.

Major Opium Alkaloids

Drugs are listed in decreasing order, from strongest to weakest in terms of
pain-controlling properties, and in increasing order for tranquilizing effectiveness:

morphine
papaverine
codeine
narcotine
narceine
thebaine

EXTRA-SPECIAL

DRUG ACCESSORIES

COCAINE CATAPULT
Two small spoons launch the cocaine directly into the nostrils. Somewhat inconvenient for club use.

SNUFF KIT, "AGATE"
Small box made of genuine leather, board made of agate, gold-colored razor blade, two gold straws, dosage vial, and spatula.

SAFE CAN
Looks and feels like an unopened soda can but is empty inside. Comes with a twist-off lid.

CAMELFLAGE
Rolled in these printed papers, joints are indistinguishable from Camel cigarettes. Until you light them, of course.

GROW BOX
Also known as a "hydro hut" or "grow tent," the construction works like a greenhouse and can be set up anywhere or placed behind a false wall. A four by four by four foot grow tent is available for around $600, complete with a 400 watt grow light, maxi light reflector, fan controller, and timer.

GRINDER
A contraption used for pulverizing marijuana. The Big-E-Grinder ("table grinder with a stylish blue design") is capable of milling the substance into the finest powder. While doing so, it also glows blue from the inside. The Grinder is also available disguised as a golf ball.

GOLDEN RAZOR BLADES
Speaking of New York in the seventies, fashion designer Wolfgang Joop once explained that cocaine was chopped with golden razor blades from Cartier. The renowned French jeweler also carried a "little matching spoon" in silver. Times have changed, according to Joop: *"These days you put the stuff in the groove of your car key."*

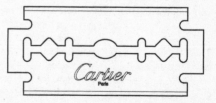

A CLASSIFICATION OF **Psychoactive**
SUBSTANCES ACCORDING TO THEIR EFFECTS

☞ <u>SEDATIVES</u>—Substances with a calming or anxiety-reducing effect. These include opiates and benzodiazepines ("benzos") like diazepam (Valium), alprazolam (Xanax), and flunitrazepam (Rohypnol).

☞ <u>STIMULANTS</u>—Substances that increase alertness or have an animating effect. Well-known examples include cocaine, amphetamine (speed), and caffeine.

☞ <u>ANTIDEPRESSIVES OR MOOD ELEVATORS</u>—Substances affecting the sensitivity of receptors in the brain. Effects are usually seen only after several days or weeks of continued use. Sudden discontinuation can cause shooting pains not unlike electric shocks, otherwise known as the "zaps."

☞ <u>DISSOCIATIVES</u>—Substances that block the consciousness from the limbic system, separating the mind from physical self-perception. Higher doses can have a narcotic effect, but may also cause hallucinations and out-of-body experiences. Examples: PCP, ketamine, the cough suppressant dextromethorphan, laughing gas, and substances derived from the plants iboga, *Salvia divinorum*, and fly agaric.

☞ <u>HALLUCINOGENS</u>—Substances that alter visual, acoustic, or haptic perception. Examples include LSD, DMT, psilocybin-containing mushrooms, mescaline, and sometimes cannabis and ecstasy (MDMA). Where the "journey" takes you depends not only on the dose, but on the user's psychological constitution and his or her expectations. Hallucinogens affect the following:

    <u>EMPATHOGENS</u>—Increase feelings of empathy and intuition.

    <u>PSYCHOTOMIMETIC</u>—Mimic psychotic symptoms. LSD research in particular has centered on its psychotomimetic properties.

    <u>EIDETICS</u>—Have a creative effect, facilitate new ideas.

    <u>ENTACTOGENS</u>—Give the user the feeling of being able to feel and get in touch with their own psychic being.

    <u>PSYCHEDELICS</u>—Trigger a euphoric, trancelike state.

    <u>PSYCHODYSLEPTICS</u>—Soften the soul.

    <u>ENTHEOGENS</u>—Awaken a feeling of godliness.

THE PRODUCTIVENESS OF POPPY

There is approximately .05 gram of opium per poppy capsule. One kilogram of opium entails the scoring and scraping of twenty thousand poppy capsules.

Harvesting one kilogram of opium requires over four thousand square feet of cultivatable land and two hundred to three hundred hours of work.

HITLER'S DRUGS

Adolf Hitler believed that alcohol, nicotine, and meat consumption formed a vicious cycle with disastrous consequences to good health. Even so, he drank aromatic digestive tonics for severe abdominal pain and intestinal gas after eating boiled foods and took up to sixteen "anti-gas" pills a day containing the neurotoxins strychnine and belladonna. Starting in 1937, perhaps even 1936, his personal physician Dr. Morell probably administered injections of the then newly-discovered methamphetamine Pervitin. From 1941 on, he received daily injections of the substance directly after waking by the "Reich injection master" as Göring called him, and doses were also administered before all important speeches and meetings. Later he would receive up to eight injections per day. Hitler also took methamphetamine-containing Vita multi tablets, made especially for him and wrapped in gold paper, ten times a day in the last year of the war. All in addition to the caffeinated Cola-Dahlmann candy that he was constantly sucking on.

The vivacity and exalted mood experienced in the beginning was followed by lethargy, depression, and fits of rage. Periods of insomnia and loss of appetite were punctuated by phases of oversleeping and excessive eating. In 1939, Hitler began to nibble the cuticles on his thumb, pointer, and middle finger on both hands, resulting in a chronic infection of the fingertips. In 1942 a Parkinson's-like tremor began in his arms and hands, for which he was treated with opiates and Testoviron, a sex hormone also popular with bodybuilders. In 1943 his neck was encrusted with infected pustules from frequent scratching. Hitler became light sensitive, lost weight, and suffered from headaches. His auditory canals bled after the failed assassination attempt on July 20, 1944. Ear, nose, and throat specialist Dr. Giesing feared a heavy sinus infection, for which he knew of only one cure: Swab the area with a 10% cocaine solution to retard swelling in the infected mucus membranes and alleviate the pain. On October 1, Hitler reacted to the cocaine swabs with pulmonary and circulatory collapse.

April 21, 1945, one day after Hitler's last birthday, Dr. Morell left the Führerbunker, taking the drug supply with him. Hitler was forced to make do with the only stimulant left: cocaine eye-drops. The drops dilated his pupils and paralyzed his eye muscles, making him so light sensitive that he could no longer step into daylight. Hitler was, when he died with Eva Braun on April 30, 1945, functionally blind.

FRIEND NUMBER 4
Drew Barrymore

The actress bared her breasts to late-night talk show host David Letterman for his forty-eighth birthday on April 12, 1995. A few weeks prior, she had received a birthday quilt from Steven Spielberg with the message *"Cover yourself up!"*—a reference to her undressing in several films and posing nude for *Playboy*. For years Drew Barrymore appeared a hopeless case. Born into a 150-year-old acting dynasty, Barrymore made her screen debut in the prophetically titled film *Altered States* at age seven and rose to child stardom in *E.T.: The Extra-Terrestrial* two years later. At fourteen she published her autobiography, *Little Girl Lost*, detailing her rapidly advancing drug career: alcohol at age eleven, cannabis at twelve, cocaine a year later, then a suicide attempt, rehab, and a "tell-it-all" memoir. For a while Barrymore languished on several blacklists despite her illustrious pedigree: *"I walked into that audition and the casting director just sat there laughing. He said: 'I can't believe you have the balls for this audition, Little Miss Drug Addict.'"* Drew Barrymore is now a successful actress and producer.

NEARLY FORGOTTEN **HOLLYWOOD** ADDICTS

In his book *Hollywood Babylon*, filmmaker and author Kenneth Anger gives a fond, tabloid-style account of sex and drug scandals from the early days of the American film industry. Some of his almost forgotten protagonists include:

★★★ OLIVE THOMAS
The actress (*The Follies Girl*) committed suicide in 1920 at the Parisian Hotel Crillon after failing to score heroin for her husband, Jack Pickford. Pickford, himself a well-known actor and often touted as the "all-American boy," was unable to answer the charges because of a nervous breakdown.

★★★ FATTY ARBUCKLE
The comedian threw one of his famous parties at the St. Francis Hotel in San Francisco. Heavily intoxicated, he disappeared with starlet Virginia Rappe and the words *"This is the chance I've waited for a long time"* into suite 1221. Guests at the party heard loud screaming; Arbuckle later reappeared at the party with her hat on his head, saying: "Go

in and get her dressed and take her to the Palace. She makes too much noise." When she would not stop yelling, Arbuckle said, *"Shut up or I'll throw you out of the window."* Rappe's companions found her in a ravaged room with her clothing in tatters, whimpering in pain. She was taken to the hospital where she bled to death from internal injuries. How Arbuckle inflicted the injuries was never proved; he was charged with rape and manslaughter but acquitted after a third trial. After the scandal, champagne bottles with his husky face on the label circulated throughout Hollywood.

★★★ WILLIAM DESMOND TAYLOR
The leading director of a Paramount Pictures subsidiary was murdered under mysterious circumstances and numerous cover-up attempts ensued. Weeks before his death, he was seen frequenting the *"queer meeting places"* of Los Angeles, where *"strange effeminate men and peculiarly masculine women"* served marijuana, opium, and morphine from a tea wagon.

★★★ WALLACE REID
The aforesaid scandals resulted in a studio crackdown, and film moguls hired Republican Will H. Hays to act as a moral watchdog. His "Doom Book" contained a list of actors with morally unsuitable conduct, and actor Wallace Reid's name stood right at the top of the list. To Paramount CEO Adolph Zukor's chagrin, Reid checked into a private sanatorium citing "exhaustion" as tabloid rumors surrounding his morphine addiction began to surface. *"Good Time Wally,"* as Kenneth Anger mused, *"took on another meaning."*

★★★ BARBARA LA MARR
"Hollywood's most glamorous, if jaded, junkie," Kenneth Anger wrote of La Marr (*Strangers of the Night*). She stashed her cocaine in a golden casket on her grand piano, her opium was *"finest grade Benares blend",* and she changed lovers "like roses." La Marr never slept more than two hours a night, having had *"better things to do,"* and died of a heroin overdose in 1926.

★★★ ALMA RUBENS
The actress streaked across Hollywood Boulevard on January 26, 1929, chased by two men and screaming, *"I'm being kidnapped!"* When they finally cornered her at a gas station, Rubens (*The Price She Paid*) stabbed one of her pursuers in the shoulder with a knife. The men were later discovered to be a medical aid and her doctor, Dr. E. W. Meyer. Rubens drifted in and out of psychiatric institutions, once assaulted a nurse, was caught with forty cubes of morphine, and died at thirty-three.

★★★ FRANCES FARMER
All she really wanted was to play Chekhov on Broadway, but the hapless actress landed in Hollywood instead. First jailed for drunk driving in 1942, Farmer's battles with both the bottle and the law only escalated from there. She was arrested in the Knickerbock-

er Hotel for violating probation, dislocated her hairdresser's jaw, lost her sweater in a nightclub, and ran topless down Sunset Strip. At the police station she listed her profession as "Cocksucker," and later explained to the judge, *"Listen, I put liquor in my milk and in my orange juice. What do you want me to do, starve to death? I drink everything I can get, including Benzedrine."* Her mother had Farmer declared legally insane and held world communism responsible.

★★★ LUPE VÉLEZ

The ex-girlfriend/wife of Gary Cooper and Johnny Weissmuller had her best acting days behind her (*Gaucho*) and was pregnant by her married lover Harald Maresch. Too Catholic to abort the child and too miserable to carry on, Vélez (called the "Mexican Spitfire") staged an opulent Mexican dinner with girlfriends, after which she went home and overdosed on Seconal to die on her flower-strewn bed. One can only assume that the funeral feast didn't agree with her; she was found the next day in her bathroom, drowned with her head in the toilet. It was an "Egyptian Chartreuse Onyx Hush-Flush Model Deluxe."

THE MOST INSIGHTFUL OF **EMINEM'S**
      ECSTASY REFLECTIONS

❝ *On the Slim Shady tour, I was fuckin' with that ecstasy shit every night, doing at least a hit every time. In the end, though, it gets hard on the body.* ❞

❝ *If I'm writing rhymes I smoke weed or take Tylenol or muscle relaxers, something to get the stories rolling. Or ecstasy. Then when I'm on stage, it's Bacardi, Hennessy, or ecstasy. I only do half a hit or maybe just a quarter. If I did a whole one I'd be gone. Eyes rolling, dribbling, all that shit.* ❞

❝ *I wrote two songs for the next album on ecstasy. Shit about bouncing off walls, going straight through 'em, falling down twenty stories. Crazy. That's what we do when I'm in the studio with Dre. We get in there, get bugged out, stay in the studio for two fuckin' days. Then you're* dead for three days. Then you wake up, pop the tape in, like, 'Let me see what I've done . . .' ❞

❝ *A couple of the songs on the new record were written on X. It exaggerates shit. Somebody will just be looking at me wrong and I'll just flip a table over, like, what the fuck are you staring at? If you're in a good mood you love everybody, but if you're in a bad mood and you got shit on your mind, you're gonna break down and shit. The hardest shit I've fucked with is X and 'shrooms.* ❞

❝ *Never take ecstasy, beer, Bacardi, weed, Pepto Bismol, Vivarin, Tums, Tagamet HB, Xanax and Valium in the same day. It makes it difficult to sleep at night.* ❞

ANIMALS ON MORPHINE

In 1939, the German chemist Hermann Römpp reported on his morphine experiments with animals. Dogs, rabbits, guinea pigs, and pigeons were narcotized, while horses, cattle, cats, sheep, and goats reacted with astonishing agitation. Cats growl. Mice on morphine cock their tails. Given a sample in their food, the crooked tail makes it possible to distinguish between mice with an absence of morphine in their systems and those who have eaten one-hundred-thousandth of a gram.

FRIEND NUMBER 5
David Bowie

With his dazzling costumes and suggestive body of work, no pop star has contributed to the glorification of drugs as much as David Bowie (born 1947). He has sung of futuristic otherworlds and isolation and looked enviable at every phase of his addiction—with the possible exception of his sometimes problematically large brown teeth. His leading role as Thomas Jerome Newton in Nicolas Roeg's *The Man Who Fell to Earth* could easily be interpreted as the portrait of a heroin junkie, though a very wealthy one. Bowie's personal drug of choice was cocaine, a favorite indulgence since the early 1970s: *"It had become such a problem that I couldn't function in any other way from day to day. I couldn't eat anything. I weighed 95 pounds or something. I am absolutely amazed that I actually survived that period."*

Bowie sang, *"It's not the side-effect of the cocaine. I'm thinking it must be love"* in *Station to Station*, the recording of which he cannot remember. By 1976 the singer had already collapsed several times due to drug overdose. An interview in which he named Adolf Hitler as one of the "first pop stars" (and compared the dictator's charisma to Mick Jagger's) was later excused by citing drug use at the time.

After rescuing his friend Iggy Pop from an L.A. psychiatric hospital (and offering a few lines of blow as a welcome gift), the two shared an apartment in Berlin's Schöneberg district. In Berlin, Bowie was the occasional lover of local celebrity transvestite Romy Haag, who later complained of Bowie's foul, cocaine-generated body odor. He kicked his coke habit before leaving the city in 1980 and later claimed that it was harder for him to quit smoking.

Recently Bowie appeared in an advertisement for French mineral water: The commercial shows him wandering through a house, where he encounters several figures embodied throughout his career: Ziggy Stardust, the Diamond Dog, and the clown from the "Ashes to Ashes" video. The second-richest entertainer in Great Britain gets a hefty paycheck for his personal flashbacks.

FRIEND NUMBER 6
Lapo Elkann

The drama on October 10, 2005, began with a short emergency call: *"Fast! Fast! At my house there is an important person that's feeling bad!"* The caller was fifty-three-year-old Donato Braco, a transsexual known as "Patrizia," the "important person" was Lapo Elkann (born 1978), Gianni Agnelli's grandson and the Fiat corporation's youngest (and maybe only) hope. Elkann was the marketing manager of the financially stricken family firm; many believed him a veritable reincarnation of his glamorous grandpa, who counted Rita Hayworth, Jackie Kennedy, and Anita Ekberg among his many conquests. Born in New York, Elkann was schooled in London and Paris, speaks five languages, worked at the Salomon Smith Barney investment bank and as Henry Kissinger's assistant; his girlfriend was a super-blonde TV showgirl. A well-known man-about-town and marketing genius, Elkann was supposed to infuse the latest Fiat models with sex appeal.

Paramedics found him on "Patrizia's" sofa in a less-than-fancy neighborhood of Turin, with twisted eyes and labored breathing. The billionaire heir and leading figure in the Agnelli family's illustrious Juventus Football Club had taken a cocktail of cocaine, alcohol, and heroin and slipped into a coma. *"We've known each other for a few months,"* stated "Patrizia" in an interview with *La Repubblica*; photographs of the transsexual in a black wig with collagen-plumped lips rapidly circulated in the Italian media, which for decades had celebrated the Agnelli clan as royalty. Elkann rang her bell before midnight, according to the police, and the two fell asleep at dawn. *"I got up at around nine and tried to wake Lapo, but he didn't show any sign of life. So I immediately called an ambulance."* After initial treatment at Mauriziano Hospital in Turin, where he lay unconscious for an entire day, Elkann checked himself into an American rehabilitation center. *"I need some time to think,"* he said. In 2007 he launched the fashion company Italia Independent.

DRUG-FREE POP MUSICIANS: FRANK ZAPPA

HOW TO TURN CUT COCAINE INTO VALUABLE **Rocks**

When cocaine isn't fine but crumbly, like little white pebbles, it is often mistakenly thought to be especially pure. One-time German drug boss Ronald Miehling explained in his book *Schneekönig (Snow King)* how dirty cocaine can be made to look like valuable "rocks":

All you need is a metallic tube about 30 mm in diameter, a car jack, a five-Mark coin, and spray acetone, a type of fingernail polish remover. The cut coke is sprayed and stirred until it looks like snow. Then it gets put in a baggie and rolled into a little sausage, and the sausage goes into the tube. The five-Mark coin, which fits in the tube exactly, goes in front, and all that is pressed against the top with the car jack using something like a ton and a half of force. You let it stand for about 30 minutes and then take the sausage out of the tube and let it dry for three, four days depending on the weather, bust it with a hammer, and you've got rocks.

HOW TO MAKE Opium SMOKABLE

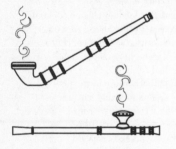

Water is poured over the opium. After standing for two days, the mixture is cooked in flat skillets and thickened to a viscous residue containing only 5% water. This is then kneaded, spread in an inch-thick layer onto a smaller pan, and held upside-down over a flame, immediately heating the substance and triggering a partial chemical decomposition. When it starts to release a strong-smelling vapor, the thus-roasted pancake is then peeled from the pan and dissolved in water again. Afterward, it is filtered for charred and insoluble components, evaporated into a syrup, whipped to a foam, and stored in partially covered jars. Fermentation occurs over the course of about three months, lending it—not unlike a cheese-making process—the characteristic bouquet of Chinese smoking opium. It is typically smoked in a thick bamboo pipe, near the end of which is a chamber with a pin-sized hole in the top. The user spears a pea-sized opium clump with a fine needle and holds it over the flame of a small, specially-designed lamp until the damp mass congeals into a tougher pill, then smushes this into the narrow opening on the pipe head. Pulling the needle free with a twisting motion, the smoker creates a tiny hole through to the bamboo stalk, inverts the pipe head over the flame, and inhales, holding the smoke in his lungs as long as possible.

U.S. PRESIDENTS

WITH ALCOHOL PROBLEMS

⭐ JOHN ADAMS (1797–1801)
Led temperance campaigns against brandy, though he himself drank a stiff, eye-opening cider every morning. Started smoking at age eight.

⭐ THOMAS JEFFERSON (1801–1809)
Critics accused him of constant drunkenness. The first draft of the Declaration of Independence was written in a bar. He claimed to drink very moderately. He also loved wine and considered himself an expert.

⭐ MARTIN VAN BUREN (1837–1841)
Nickname "Blue Whisky Van." He could consume enormous amounts of alcohol without ever getting drunk.

⭐ FRANKLIN PIERCE (1853–1857)
"What will I do after my presidency? There's nothing left to do but get drunk." He died of liver cirrhosis.

⭐ JAMES BUCHANAN (1857–1861)
A wealthy bachelor with a considerable appetite. He had a very high tolerance and ordered small bottles of champagne to be delivered to the White House.

⭐ ANDREW JOHNSON (1865–1869)
Had three whiskeys before his vice-presidential inauguration, slurred, and talked rather incoherently. Later became a Prohibition advocate.

⭐ ULYSSES S. GRANT (1869–1877)
Joined the Sons of Temperance with no success. Also smoked up to twenty cigars per day. His throat cancer was swabbed with cocaine to ease the pain, and he became an addict.

⭐ CHESTER ARTHUR (1881–1885)
Loved fine wines and liqueur for dessert.

⭐ GROVER CLEVELAND (1885–1889/1893)
Rumors persisted during his second term that he was a heavy drinker and abused his wife. He could not be anesthetized with ether during his bout with palate cancer, as alcohol had made him resistant to it. Cocaine was used instead.

⭐ WARREN HARDING (1921–1923)
Drank whiskey on the sly, despite Prohibition laws. Gambled away the White House porcelain at poker.

⭐ GEORGE W. BUSH (2001–2009)
Former alcoholic, though medical reports show that he has been abstinent since 1986. In his first presidential campaign, Bush explained that he has not taken cocaine since 1992, later he said not since 1974. Unlike the president, everyone in his administration is required to sign a security clearance stating that they have taken no drugs past the age of eighteen.

AFGHANISTAN VERSUS COLOMBIA

After dropping to an all-time low after the 2001 Taliban opium ban, Afghanistan is once again the world's leading supplier for the heroin market. Colombia remains number one in cocaine production. Some numbers:

AFGHANISTAN
Net opium poppy cultivation ⟫→ 165,000 hectares
Percentage of global cultivation ⟫→ 82%
Potential production of opium ⟫→ 6,100 metric tons
Percentage of global cultivation ⟫→ 92%
Number of persons involved in opium cultivation ⟫→ 2.9 million
Percentage of total population ⟫→ 12.6%
Average farm-gate price of dry opium at harvest time ⟫→ $125 per kilogram
Total farm-gate value of opium production ⟫→ $0.76 billion
Percentage of GDP ⟫→ 11%
Total export value of opium to neighboring countries ⟫→ $3.1 billion
Percentage of GDP ⟫→ 46%
Per capita gross income of opium growing farmers ⟫→ $260
Afghanistan GDP per capita ⟫→ $290
Indicative gross income from opium per hectare ⟫→ $4,600
Indicative gross income from wheat per hectare ⟫→ $530

COLOMBIA
Net coca cultivation ⟫→ 78,000 hectares
Potential production of cocaine ⟫→ 610 metric tons
Percentage of world cocaine production ⟫→ 62%
Average farm-gate price of coca paste ⟫→ $879 per kilogram
Average cocaine price (wholesale) ⟫→ $1,762 per kilogram   Source: UN 2007 World Drug Report

DRUG TREATMENT

PER MILLION INHABITANTS IN 2005

Americas	3,674
Oceania	2,288
Europe	847
Asia	117
Africa	29
Global average	696

ANIMALS ON CANNABIS

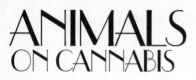

MICE

✸ A male mouse will show increased sexual interest in females, though at higher doses he gets clumsier and can barely mount the female mouse. Eventually the male mouse will yawn and shift his attention to himself—bathes, licks his penis.

RABBITS

✸ When animals of the same weight are given the same dose of a substance, some will show drastic disturbances and others no reaction at all: These animals frequently slide all four legs away from their bodies until they are lying flat on their stomachs. Legs are held in grotesque positions and hang from the body as if dislocated. Often the animals will lie on one side, panting. Righting reflexes are compromised; instead of standing upright they lean their bodies in any direction. Quick reflexes are undisturbed when stimulated.

DOGS

✸ Begin by slightly wagging the lowered head. The wagging gradually moves over the entire body, eventually becoming so strong that the animal nearly falls over. Dogs will often stand still in one spot, hopping to the side now and then when their balance is threatened. Sometimes the hind legs or spine will buckle even when the animal is not sitting down. When they do attempt to sit, it is achieved only with great difficulty, sinking down bit by bit, down through to the hindquarters. The forelimbs are stiffly splayed in front of their bodies until the torso rests on the floor, thighs gliding apart until the animal is lying flat. The head lowers, getting startled every time it touches the floor. These animals show a jumpy response to calling or hand clapping; aggressive dogs become clingy and affectionate.

GOLDFISH

✸ First appear dead in the water. After half an hour they begin to convulse; bit by bit the jerky movements give way to normal swimming.

WHICH ALCOHOL IS THE MOST FATTENING?

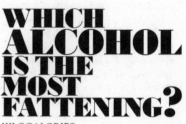

KILOCALORIES
PER GRAM OF ALCOHOL:

Whiskey, pure (45%)	6.8
Vodka, pure (40%)	7.0
Cabinet white wine (dry)	8.0
Red wine (heavy)	8.1
Champagne (brut)	8.2
Red wine (light)	8.8
Hefeweizen (5.7%)	10.7
Pilsner (4.9%)	11.0
Sparkling wine (sweet)	12.1
Vodka tonic	12.9
Caipirinha	20.5
Beck's Alcohol Free	60.0

THE GREATEST

DRUG POPES

OF GERMANY AND SWITZERLAND

WALTER BENJAMIN (1892–1940)

♣ The essayist was unconvinced that his occasional hashish experiments in the late 1920s had revealed any hidden truths in themselves, but did feel that they allowed him to explore the illusive surface of things. *"The opium smoker or hashish eater experiences the power of imbibing at a glance a hundred sites from a single spot."* This is the so-called "profane illumination." If experienced permanently as an addiction, it can make an individual "more suitable" for the daily struggle for existence. Addicts just look better, because *"unkindness, fanaticism about being correct, and pharasaism"* have disappeared. This *"intensifying attractiveness"* was for Benjamin a primary motive of addiction.

GOTTFRIED BENN (1886–1956)

♣ As a military doctor during World War I, Gottfried Benn had unlimited access to drugs. He took cocaine and later the painkiller *"pyramidone, à la carte and in heaps."* In 1943, when he rarely or never touched narcotics, the poet and essayist acknowledged being high as the "prime cause" of life: *"From hidden centers, from the depths it emerges: to rest, to move no more—: withdrawal, regression, aphasia. Hours are filled with the satisfied desire to drift along as formless life. To call this animalistic is to be mistaken: this process is far below the animals, below the reflexes, it is near roots, chalk, and stone.*

"Potent brains are not strengthened through milk but through alkaloids. An organ of such small size and great vulnerability, which not only approached the pyramids and gamma-rays, lions and icebergs, but created and invented them, cannot be watered like a forget-me-not; it will find its own supplies."

Benn's recommendation in the latter phases of World War II: *"Rather than give it to bomber pilots and explorers, Pervitin [methamphetamine], could be purposefully used in high schools and colleges to promote cerebral oscillations."*

ALBERT HOFMANN (1906–2008)

♣ Hard at work in Switzerland's Sandoz Laboratories (now Novartis), the pharmaceutical chemist was actually trying to come up with a new blood circulation therapy when, in 1938, he accidentally synthesized LSD for the first time. Animal laboratory tests showed no reactions, but in 1943 Hofmann re-created the solution out of a gut feeling that the substance must have some effect and unintentionally came into contact with it. On his bike ride home, he began to experience a hallucinogenic trip. Hofmann compared his discovery to the simultaneous discovery of nuclear power: *"One could assume that these coincidences have been put into play by the Weltgeist ('World Spirit')."* Though he has continued to take LSD into a ripe old age, he also warns of its dangers and has expressed his disappointment with both the excesses of the 1960s and the subsequent ban on LSD.

ERNST JÜNGER (1895–1998)

The adventurous son of a food chemist joined the French Foreign Legion in 1913 and fought in World War I as a volunteer. By World War II he could only put up with it as an impassive bystander. Then the search for inner adventures began: He tried hallucinogenic drugs. Having been invited by Albert Hofmann in 1951 to experiment with the new drug LSD, Jünger noted: *"Wine has already changed much, has brought new gods and a new humanity with it. But wine is to the new substances as classical physics is to modern physics. These things should only be tried in small circles."*

In his novel *Besuch auf Godenholm* (*Visit to Godenholm*) Jünger describes the LSD experience in his characteristically bombastic style: *"Myriads of molecules observed the harmony. Here the laws no longer acted under the veil of appearance; matter was so delicate and weightless that it clearly reflected them. How simple and cogent everything was."* While the hippies made drug consumption synonymous with youth, the seventy-five-year-old supported the legalization of drugs for seniors in the 1970s. So close to death already, they would have nothing to lose but boredom.

WOLFGANG NEUSS (1923–1989)

The German World War II enlisted man and trained butcher from Breslau shot off his own finger so that he could be sent to the military hospital, where he first gained a reputation as a joke teller. After the war Neuss became the most famous cabaret artist in Germany, constantly on the move, thanks to a steady stream of stimulants, sleeping pills, and alcohol. In the seventies he switched to cannabis and psychedelics—*"I smoked the rope that would hang me"*—and spent the majority of days sitting quietly on the floor of his underground dwelling.

Legend has it that he typically smoked at least twenty strong joints per day and once, after taking twenty trips of strong acid,

WHAT

HELPS AGAINST

Coughing
Bad mood
Aggression
Anxiety
Pain
Sleep disorders
Diarrhea
Obesity
Breathing
  problems
Lying

quietly remained in the sitting position. Neuss eventually became a prophet to the '68 generation; he was Germany's last hippie, and declared: *"Perpetual bliss is something only an addict can have."*

For Neuss, culture can be found wherever ecstasy is, *"and if we want to know where this war frenzy came from in the thirties then we have to look at what the ecstasy was up to in the 1910s and twenties. And what do we see there: We see the chieftans of World War I who took cocaine and opium by the spoonful, we see the whole culture scene, the Brechts, Tucholskys, the Dadaists, either they themselves were getting high or they were surrounded by people who were high. (. . .) and what does the little non-thinker person notice when he takes drugs and expands his consciousness: He suddenly gets that 'man, we're all the same.' The whole world is spiritually connected and whatever I'm thinking now will be done tomorrow. Not by me, but somebody else will do it—but the Nazis, the nature ecstatics, Goebbels, Hitler, and his doctor Morell didn't get that far. They just caught a glimpse of this total awareness that we're all the same and immediately tried to implement it, so to speak: Yes, we're all the same! Yes, we've all got to be blond! All that nonsense. So that's why I'm saying that fascism is basically drug history gone wrong, dealing with ecstasy in the wrong way."*

NINA HAGEN (BORN 1955)

✠ *"Cocaine is a very stupid, incredibly physically and spiritually corrosive drug,"* she once said in an interview, though she would have liked to eat a piece of a mushroom with GDR president Erich Honecker in drag—then he would have seen *"that the trees can dance."* She took Dormutil, a sleep medication popular as a party drug, in an East Berlin garden and experienced her first French kiss. At nineteen she took LSD for the first time to "find God" and heard a gentle male voice say, *"Nina, I am here. I will help you."* After her move to the West and a very successful debut album, Hagen became romantically involved with Dutch musician and junkie Herman Brood, who later committed suicide, and with guitarist Ferdinand Karmelk, who allegedly crumbled heroin into her joints. Her song "African Reggae" is a hymn of praise to pot smoking: *"It smells so fine, watch out you don't get busted. 'Cause they're after you, you old stoner. So what if their world is going to pot from alcoholism."*

Nina Hagen is not only an active Drug Pope, she is also an ambassador of masturbation, ufology, the peace movement, animal rights, vocal acrobatics, and Buddhism.

HEROIN OR COCAINE?

In a comparison test, one group of rats was given heroin and another cocaine. After one month, the heroin rats showed a typical addict's daily routine: take drugs, eat, walk around, sleep, take more drugs, sleep. All of the cocaine rats were dead.

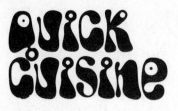

EAZ-Y COOKIES

Ingredients
- ⊙ Cream-filled chocolate cookies
- ⊙ Grass as desired

Preparation
- ⊙ Remove the top half of the cookie.
- ⊙ Crumble the weed inside.
- ⊙ Replace the cookie top.
- ⊙ Microwave on High for 30 seconds.

PEANUT BUTTER SANDWICH

Ingredients
- ⊙ Two pieces of toast
- ⊙ Peanut butter
- ⊙ Marijuana as desired

Preparation
- ⊙ Smear peanut butter on both pieces of toast (only on one side of each).
- ⊙ Crumble marijuana onto the peanut butter.
- ⊙ Place the other slice of toast on top.
- ⊙ Grill until slightly crisp.
- ⊙ Enjoy warm.

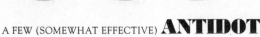

A FEW (SOMEWHAT EFFECTIVE) **ANTIDOTES**

FLUMAZENIL helps against anxiolytics of the benzodiazepine class such as Valium (Diazepam) or Versed (Midazolam). The substance binds to the same receptors, reversing the effects. The comatose user wakes up with a jolt.

DISULFIRAM doesn't help in cases of alcohol overdose but prevents you from drinking it in the first place. Disulfiram blocks acetaldehyde dehydrogenase, an enzyme responsible for metabolizing alcohol. Taking it and drinking

even tiny amounts of alcohol will cause flushed skin, nausea, and headaches.

BETA-BLOCKERS cannot reverse the effects of cocaine or speed but can soften certain symptoms such as heart palpitations.

NALOXON AND NALTREXONE are effective against heroin and other opiates. They are injected into the comatose user—seconds later his eyes snap open and he's making small talk.

DRUGS FOUND IN NATURE

DEADLY NIGHTSHADE, BELLADONNA

● All parts of this nightshade plant, particularly its shiny black berries, contain both hyoscyamine and scopolamine. Hyoscyamine is a hallucinogen, and scopolamine causes apathy. The ancient Greeks reported incidents of nightshade berry being mixed into wine. Because it also dilates the pupils, the substance was also dropped into the eyes as a cosmetic. There is a fine line between the plant's mind-altering and deadly effects.

ALRAUNE, MANDRAKE

● Another nightshade plant with effects similar to belladonna. Mandrake root can sometimes resemble a human face, making it especially popular as a magic-bearing ingredient in Europe. The Catholic mystic Hildegard von Bingen believed that mandrake was the seat of the devil. Before being used as a remedy for sexual desire, for example, it would have to be soaked in pure spring water.

HENBANE

● Also contains scopolamine and especially large amounts of hyoscyamine. Witches in the Middle Ages were said to have used henbane to make "flying ointment," which they would rub over their entire bodies. The solution was especially well absorbed by vaginal mucous membranes—upon which they would ride away on their flying brooms.

Henbane seeds were also often scattered on the ovens of bathhouses at the time; the steam was especially relaxing, making it easier for men to "encounter" women in the bathtubs. Until the German Purity Laws were passed in 1516, henbane was often used as a buzz-enhancing flavoring ingredient in beer. Henbane also leads to dry mouth and therefore causes thirst. Both the city of Pilsen and Pilsner beer are supposedly named after *Bilsenkraut*, the German word for henbane.

DATURA

● A nightshade plant with more of the hallucinogenic hyoscyamine. The Aztecs gave their human sacrifices datura to make them more compliant. In India, datura was also known as "Shiva's head of hair," referring to the god of destruction.

BRUGMANSIA

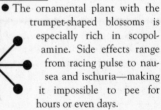

● The ornamental plant with the trumpet-shaped blossoms is especially rich in scopolamine. Side effects range from racing pulse to nausea and ischuria—making it impossible to pee for hours or even days.

EPHEDRA

● Ephedra contains the alkaloid ephedrine, which raises body temperature and blood pressure and induces euphoria. Ephedrine is one of the basic ingredients for synthesizing methamphetamine. Up until its FDA ban in 2004, the substance was widely available in U.S. pharmacies as a weight-loss supplement, known to take the edge off of hunger and boost metabolism. Mormon pioneers used to drink an ephedra-containing brew called "Mormon tea" as a replacement for caffeine, which was forbidden by the church.

ST. JOHN'S WORT
● St. John's wort grows almost everywhere in the world, and extracts of St. John's wort have been used medicinally since antiquity. The plant is a mood elevator and has antidepressive effects, though it also makes the skin more sensitive to light. Farmers consider it a noxious weed.

HOPS
● Hop belongs to the cannabis, or hemp, family. The female buds, also known as "hops," contain lupulin and have a calming effect. Though primarily used as a flavoring agent in beer, the plant has a long history of medicinal use as well. Pillows filled with dried hops were once used to treat sleep disorders. Hops can also be smoked.

CASTOREUM, BEAVER SECRETIONS
● The two 20-to-100-gram heavy glandular sacks located between the beaver's anus and genitals contain the brownish, resinlike beaver secretions. The scent resembles valeriana; the taste is intense, bitter, and aromatic. Beaver secretions were used as a remedy against cramping, hysterical fits, and nervousness until the

nineteenth century. In Greco-Roman antiquity, they were applied in the treatment of epilepsy. Demand for the substance was so high that beavers became endangered. Castoreum is now used only homeopathically and in a few aphrodisiac perfumes.

PSILOCYBIN MUSHROOMS
● Mushrooms that contain psilocin or psilocybin are similar to LSD in effect. Optical and acoustic perception is intensified and, in higher doses, also distorted. Hallucinations result. Unlike LSD, the effects flatten out after only a few hours. The most common type of psilo mushroom is *Psilocybe semilanceata* (Liberty cap)—a small mushroom with a pointy, brownish to olive-yellow, somewhat slimy head, finely striped at the edge. It sometimes has a bluish to greenish tint. The gills are violet-gray to deep purple-brown with white-frosted blades. Caution: psilocybin mushrooms found growing on waste wood are easily confused with *Gallerina* variety mushrooms (Death cap, Destroying angel), a species that contains deadly amounts of Alpha-amanitin toxins. Even purchased mushrooms have their disadvantages. Sometimes the so-called "psilos" are just regular dried mushrooms spiked with a little cheap LSD.

MANROOT, WILD CUCUMBER
● The wild cucumber is commonly found in western North America. The spiny fruit contains four large hallucinogenic seeds. Effects can be felt after ingesting only one seed. Hallucinogenic properties

are strongest in the spring, when the fruit is not yet completely ripe.

LOBELIA, INDIAN TOBACCO, PUKEWEED

● The leaves of this herbaceous bell-flower have a tobaccolike taste, but their euphoria-inducing effects are more like those of marijuana than nicotine. Lobelia can also be consumed in the form of a tea—best with a sober stomach.

HAWAIIAN BABY WOODROSE

● The creeping vine can reach a height of up to thirty feet. Its unripe seeds (Hawaiian babies) contain Lysergic acid amide (LSA), similar to LSD in both chemical structure and psychedelic properties. Its mind-altering effects can be felt after ingesting only three seeds. Hawaiian baby woodrose also contains other toxic alkaloids that can cause nausea. Some users recommend removing the seeds' white, fuzzy coating with a toothbrush; others swear by ginger to ease stomach discomfort.

MORNING GLORY

● Some types of this creeping vine (particularly Pearly Gates and Heavenly Blue) also contain LSA. Users will often grind the seeds beforehand in a pepper grinder to release their full potential.

CALIFORNIA POPPY

● Though the yellow-gold state flower of California is opium-free, it does contain other calming and pain-relieving alkaloids. When smoked it produces a mild high that lasts for around thirty minutes.

WILD LETTUCE

● This wild, prickly lettuce is a particularly bitter-tasting variety. Its leaves and the milky substance contained in the stalks have calming, pain-relieving properties, higher doses of which can lead to headaches, sweating, and dizziness. European doctors once used wild lettuce as a substitute for opium and in the treatment of nymphomania. Achieving an opium-like consistency is as easy as putting the vegetable in a mixer, then allowing the juice to sit in the sun until the water evaporates, leaving only a gummy, greenish-brown residue.

WATER LILY, LOTUS

● Both blue and white lotus blossoms contain nuciferine, a soothing, anxiety-relieving, mood-brightening alkaloid. Ancient Egyptians were known to soak the flowers in wine, and Homer writes in *The Odyssey*: "And whosoever of them ate of the honey-sweet fruit of the lotus, had no longer any wish to bring back word or to return, but there they were fain to abide among the Lotus-eaters, feeding on the lotus, and forgetful of their homeward way. These men, therefore, I brought back perforce to the ships, weeping, and dragged them beneath the benches and bound them fast in the hollow ships; and I bade the rest of my trusty comrades to embark with speed on the swift ships, lest perchance anyone should eat of the lotus and forget his homeward way." Advanced users dabble at straining the plants' rhizomes.

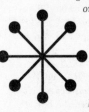

FRIEND NUMBER 7
Calvin Klein

"If there's something I want to do, nothing stops me," he once
said. In his heyday, the fashion designer would stay at Studio
54 until it closed to help the waiters count change before
heading to the Flamingo (a gay after-hours club)—then it
was on to the Mineshaft, where men were openly having sex.
He hung out with porn actors and invited hustlers home, feeding
them cocaine and Quaaludes (apparently his own drugs of choice,
aside from vodka) and knew how to translate his erotic obsessions into
mass marketing: His advertising featuring perfectly formed young men in
underwear helped to redefine masculinity and made him a fortune. In 1986 Klein (born
1942) married his assistant Kelly Rector, whom Klein greeted at his job interview with
the only modestly flirtatious line, *"The last thing I need is another pretty face with an
opinion."* Actually, it was exactly what he needed. The AIDS crisis had made his formerly flamboyant lifestyle seem somewhat out of fashion. The designer never was really
able to put the old days behind him, though; in 1988 he checked into rehab and joined
Alcoholics Anonymous. In 2003 he attended a New York Knicks basketball game and at
some point staggered onto the court to make conversation with the players.

PSYCHOTROPIC FISH

Some species of fish produce hallucinogenic substances. U.S. marine biologists
discovered the "dream fish" (*Kyphosus fuscus*) near the Norfolk Islands in 1960. The
indigenous people living there believed that eating the fish caused nightmares. Joe
Roberts, a *National Geographic* photographer, decided to eat some of the cooked meat
from the fish. Afterward he reported, *"It was pure science fiction."* Roberts said that he
saw (nonexistent) new car models and monuments to the first journey into space.

TYPES OF PSYCHOTROPIC FISH:
BLUEFISH (*Kyphosus cinerascens*)—Indonesia
BRASSY CHUB (*Kyphosus vaigiensis*)—Indonesia
CORAL GROUPER (*Epinephelus corallicola*)—Pacific Ocean
FLATHEAD MULLET (*Mugil cephalus*)—Tropical and subtropical waters worldwide
GOATFISH (*Upeneus arge*)—Indonesia
GOLDEN GOATFISH (*Mulloidichthys samoensis*)—Indonesia
MULLET FISH (*Neomyxus chaptali*)—Indonesia
RABBITFISH (*Saganus oramin*)—Indonesia, West Africa
SERGEANT MAJOR (*Abudefduf septemfasciatus*)—Pacific Ocean, Africa

HOW AND WHERE
YOU CAN GET IT

THROUGH THE SKIN

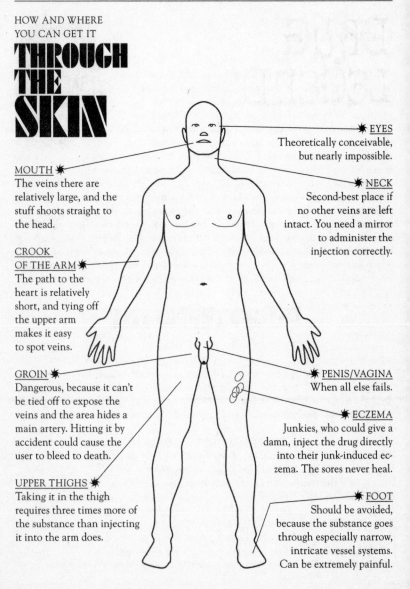

EYES
Theoretically conceivable,
but nearly impossible.

MOUTH
The veins there are
relatively large, and the
stuff shoots straight to
the head.

NECK
Second-best place if
no other veins are left
intact. You need a mirror
to administer the
injection correctly.

**CROOK
OF THE ARM**
The path to the
heart is relatively
short, and tying off
the upper arm
makes it easy
to spot veins.

GROIN
Dangerous, because it can't
be tied off to expose the
veins and the area hides a
main artery. Hitting it by
accident could cause the
user to bleed to death.

PENIS/VAGINA
When all else fails.

ECZEMA
Junkies, who could give a
damn, inject the drug directly
into their junk-induced eczema. The sores never heal.

UPPER THIGHS
Taking it in the thigh
requires three times more of
the substance than injecting
it into the arm does.

FOOT
Should be avoided,
because the substance goes
through especially narrow,
intricate vessel systems.
Can be extremely painful.

DRUG LEGENDS

ADOLPHINE

◆ Eli Lilly first brought methadone on the U.S. market in 1947 under the trade name Dolophine, or Dolphine for short. The substance was known as "Adolphine" in seventies New York street slang; Scientologists in particular spread rumors that the medication was named after "Adolph" Hitler. Actually, the word is a simple word compound, derived from the Latin *dolor* (pain) and *finis* (end).

ANTI-HEMP MAFIA

◆ In his book *The Emperor Wears No Clothes*, Jack Herer explains how the 1937 hemp business ban was an oil industry conspiracy to hinder the development of hemp-derived biodiesel.

ASSASSINS

◆ The Persian scholar Hassan-i Sabbah (1034–1124) brought young men to Alamut, his fortress located high in the mountains of what is now northern Iran. Behind the fort was a paradise garden, hidden from view by cliffs. Hassan-i Sabbah drugged the youths with opium and hashish and carried them sleeping to the garden, which was filled with pretty girls, so that when they awoke, they sincerely believed that they were in paradise. Promising a return to this heavenly place, he emboldened the lads against their fear of death and persuaded them to carry out his murder plots in the name of bringing Ismaili Shiite Muslims to power. The modern suicide assassin type was born.

COCAINE SPRAY CANS

◆ The cocaine-related substance procaine is allegedly available in aerosol spray cans in the United States, and with a little time and patience it is supposedly possible to isolate the substance at home. The myth is taken up in Philip K. Dick's novel *A Scanner Darkly*.

NEPALESE TEMPLE BALLS

◆ Rumors of highly potent white hashish balls known only to certain Indian and Nepalese monks have circulated since the 1970s. "Nepalese balls" or "temple shit" hit the European market in the mid-seventies, though actually it was a synthetically manufactured variant of the cannabis active ingredient THC, mixed with alfalfa flour as a carrier agent.

FLASHBACKS

◆ Drug opponents are constantly reporting on the danger of flashbacks recurring days or weeks later, the "boomerang high" that begins again without warning. The phenomenon is connected to the use of only one drug, namely LSD. Cases of this are in fact extremely rare, even more seldom than the so-called "atypical progression," or horror trip. New research suggests that flashbacks are more likely caused by preexisting psychological disorders such as post-traumatic stress disorder or schizophrenia.

JOHNNY POT
✦ On October 15, 1968, the FBI launched a large-scale manhunt in search of a phantom: A certain Johnny Pot was on the loose, wandering the country and dispensing cannabis wherever he went. The nationwide alert was also broadcast on television—with no photo and no luck apprehending the fugitive.

DRY ICE
✦ The effectiveness of low-grade hashish and marijuana is supposedly boosted with the help of dry ice (frozen carbon dioxide). Both are placed in a perforated shoebox and deposited in the refrigerator overnight, effectively transforming the nonpsychoactive CBD into potent THC.

MORPHINE IN FOOD
✦ Allegedly the morphine level found in poppy seeds has increased dramatically in recent years, which explains why dishes like lemon poppy-seed cake or certain noodles can be so addictive. The attributed cause is a newly introduced harvesting technique that squeezes the capsules, releasing a milky substance that contaminates the seeds.

BULLETPROOF WITH COCAINE
✦ A rumor in early 1900s America claimed that blacks gain such incredible strength from using cocaine that they become impervious to shots from a 32-caliber pistol, which at the time was commonly used by police. This was supposedly the reason that many police stations in the South switched to 38-caliber pistols.

CRUSHED GLASS IN COCAINE
✦ A few dealers purportedly cut cocaine with crushed glass, causing tiny cuts on the nasal lining, and apparently allowing the drug to work just that much better.

THIRD REICH ALIVE
✦ When the album *Autobahn* came out in the mid-seventies, American music journalist Lester Bangs (1948–1982) saw the future of rock in the German electronic band Kraftwerk: *"It's been taken over by the Germans and the machines."* Paving the way for the victory was the German discovery of amphetamine: *"The Germans invented 'speed' for the Americans . . . to destroy themselves with, thus leaving the world of pop music open for ultimate conquest."* And: *"The Reich never died. It just reincarnated in American archetypes ground out by hollow-eyed, jerky-fingered mannikins locked into their typewriters and guitars like rhinoceroses copulating."* As for the Germans themselves, Kraftwerk only goes to show that they were way past needing the drug to transform themselves into machines.

URINAL CAKE POPPERS
✦ The German author Christian Kracht claims that urine and toilet deodorizer blocks spontaneously combine to form the sex drug poppers. All you have to do is lean your face into the urinal's toi-

let lolly after relieving yourself. Taken together, the ammonia from urine and the deodorizing chlorine nitrate cause a strong shudder down the spine, the so-called "piss shiver."

BANANADINE

✦ It is sometimes whispered that banana peels, when smoked, can be high inducing. This is, however, a completely useless practice. Rumors that banana peels contain a psychoactive agent called "bananadine" were a parody spread by freaks and hippies as a reaction to the ban on hashish. In the *Anarchist Cookbook*, author William Powell explains how the fruit contains traces of "musa sapientum bananadine," a mild, short-acting psychedelic. According to the author, the advantage of this method is that it's legal:

◆ *Obtain 15 lb. of ripe yellow bananas.*
◆ *Peel the bananas and eat the fruit. Save the skins.*
◆ *With a sharp knife, scrape off the insides of the skins and save the scraped material.*
◆ *Put all scraped material in a large pot and add water. Boil for three to four hours until it has attained a solid paste consistency.*
◆ *Spread this paste on cookie sheets and dry it in an oven for about 20–30 minutes. This will result in a fine black powder (bananadine). Usually one will feel the effects of bananadine after smoking three or four cigarettes.*

The Donovan song "Mellow Yellow" was understood as a hymn to the banana high, and the band Country Joe and the Fish reportedly passed out banana joints to audience members. Andy Warhol made fun of this with his cover art for the first Velvet Underground album; members of his New York circle thought of hippies as "scruffy, dirty people" (John Cale). Powell has since disowned his work: *"The book, in many respects, was a misguided product of my adolescent anger at the prospect of being drafted and sent to Vietnam to fight in a war that I did not believe in."*

CANNIBAL HIGH

✦ Human blood, brains, and spinal fluid contain traces of the hallucinogen DMT. Schizophrenics reportedly have a higher concentration of it in their systems. The story "The Blood of a Wig" by Terry Southern is about a man who gets high on a schizophrenic's blood.

MOLDY AFGHAN

✦ Hashish with a layer of mold on top is supposedly especially potent. Nonsense: It sat too long in a damp plastic baggie and causes nausea.

FEDERAL LSD PRIESTS

✦ Drug priests such as Ken Kesey and Timothy Leary were, by an interesting double-spy theory, taken for federal CIA agents, on a mission to introduce LSD into everyday life and win acceptance for government mind control experiments.

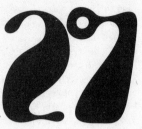

DEAD AT

✚ BRIAN JONES (2/28/1942–7/3/1969)
The Rolling Stones founding member
drowned in his own swimming pool
under the influence of drugs and alcohol.
On his deathbed, Frank Thorogood,
Jones's former workman, confessed to
murdering Jones.

✚ JIMI HENDRIX
(11/27/1942–9/18/1970)
Hendrix cancelled his depressing 1970
European tour and withdrew to London
to German girlfriend Monika Danne-
mann. He took sleeping pills and drank
alcohol, then died in his own vomit.

✚ ALAN WILSON (7/4/1943–9/3/1970)
Guitarist and singer with the blues-rock
band Canned Heat. Died of a heroin
overdose.

✚ JANIS JOPLIN (1/19/1943–10/4/1970)
*"You've gotta be crazy to take drugs if you
can get drunk on Southern Comfort instead,"* the singer supposedly said, but she
died at the Landmark Hotel in L.A. from
an overdose of heroin with fourteen holes
in her arm. In keeping with the singer's
wishes, two hundred friends drank away
the $2,500 in cash that Joplin left behind
at a party in San Anselmo, California.

✚ JIM MORRISON (12/8/1943–7/3/1971)
The Doors frontman was found dead in
his bathtub in Paris. Though the official
cause of death was "heart failure," there
are countless theories about the real
cause (suicide, kidnapped by the CIA,
murdered by a witch). Presumably Morrison died of an overdose of heroin delivered to him by Jean de Breteuil, a playboy
and his girlfriend Pamela Courson's lover.
She later claimed that Morrison thought
he was taking cocaine. Courson herself
died in 1974, also at the age of twenty-
seven, of a heroin overdose.

✚ RON "PIGPEN" MCKERNAN
(9/8/1945–3/8/1973)
The founding member of the Grateful
Dead was a heavy alcoholic. He died of a
gastrointestinal hemorrhage.

✚ DAVE ALEXANDER
(6/3/1947–2/10/1975)
Bassist for the Stooges. Died of a lung
infection linked to excessive drug consumption.

✚ GARY THAIN (5/15/1948–12/8/1975)
Played bass for Uriah Heep before being
kicked out because of his drug addiction.
Died from an overdose of heroin.

✝ JEAN-MICHEL BASQUIAT
(12/22/1960–8/12/1988)
The New York painter died of a heroin overdose. A little-known fact: He also recorded a hip-hop record.

✝ KURT COBAIN (2/20/1967–4/5/1994)
Nirvana singer and guitarist Cobain shot himself in his Seattle home following a long struggle with heroin addiction. Next to his body was a suicide note that read "It's better to burn out than to fade away," a line from the Neil Young song "My My, Hey Hey."

✝ KRISTEN PFAFF
(5/26/1967–6/16/1994)
The one-time bass guitarist for Hole died of a heroin overdose shortly after a fight with bandleader Courtney Love.

FRIEND NUMBER 8

Jack Nicholson

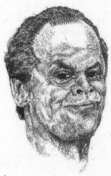

"The only reason that cocaine is such a rage today is that people are too dumb and too lazy to get themselves together and roll a joint" the three-time Oscar winner Nicholson (born 1937) said in the drug-drenched late seventies, though he has also admitted to trying every drug imaginable. With films like *The Trip* (screenplay), *Psych-Out* (leading role), and *Easy Rider* (supporting role), the star has actively glorified drug use. A key member of the New Hollywood ratpack, Nicholson's drug of choice was cocaine. He kept two qualities at home: one for visitors and acquaintances, and the better one for friends and sex partners. *"Chicks dig it sexually,"* he explained to *Playboy*, rather scientifically: *"The property of the drug is, while it numbs some areas, it inflames the mucous membranes such as in a lady's genital region. That's the real attraction of it."* He learned from Errol Flynn that *"putting a little cocaine on the top of your dick might act like an aphrodisiac."*

In his book *The Hollywood Connection*, former dealer Rayce Newman describes how Nicholson would order a few call girls from Madame Alex or Heidi Fleiss. Usually he would ask for two, three at a time, regardless of whether Rebecca Broussard, the mother of his children, was home. Angelica Houston, his lover of many years, commented, *"Of course drugs were fun. And that's what's so stupid about anti-drug campaigns: They don't admit that. I can't say I feel particularly scarred or lessened by my experimentation with drugs. They've gotten a very bad name."* When Jack Nicholson played a gangster boss in Martin Scorsese's *The Departed*, he insisted on adding a rather impressive sex toy and a huge amount of cocaine to his performance. *"I can still cause trouble,"* he said.

#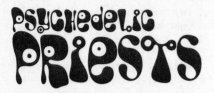

ALDOUS HUXLEY (1894–1963)

◉ Every mind was part of a universal spirit to writer Aldous Huxley, but survival was a matter of restricting, reducing, filtering the brain. The filter could be temporarily removed with the help of LSD or mescaline. On his deathbed and unable to speak, the cancer sufferer asked his wife for LSD in writing. She granted his request and Huxley died the following morning.

ALLEN GINSBERG (1926–1997)

◉ Tripping on psilocybin in 1960, the Beatnik poet envisioned a new age in which love and peace would reign on earth. Many world leaders would also need to be turned on to the experience so that they too could see the vision. A dream took flight: World peace was only a matter of putting LSD in the drinking water.

DR. OSCAR JANIGER (1918–2001)

◉ The Los Angeles–based psychiatrist, a cousin of Allen Ginsberg, studied the effects of LSD on creativity in the late 1950s and early 1960s. Study participants included André Previn, James Coburn, Lord Buckley, Anaïs Nin, and Jack Nicholson.

CARY GRANT (1904–1986)

◉ Nearly sixty years old, actor Cary Grant underwent LSD psychotherapy under Oscar Janiger. He took LSD on a weekly basis over the course of one year and raved, *"I have been born again. I have been through a psychiatric experience which has completely changed me. I was horrendous. I had to face things about myself which I never admitted, which I didn't know were there. Now I know that I hurt every woman I ever loved. I was an utter fake, a self-opinionated bore, a know-all who knew very little. I found I was hiding behind all kinds of defenses, hypocrisies, and vanities. I had to get rid of them layer by layer. The moment when your conscious meets your subconscious is a hell of a wrench. With me there came a day when I saw the light . . . Every day now is wonderful."*

Afterward Grant, who had often been taken for a homosexual, conceived his first child.

WILLIAM S. BURROUGHS (1914–1997)

◉ Burroughs was primarily a heroin junkie, but in a 1964 essay published in *LSD: The Consciousness-Expanding Drug*, he asserted that hallucinogens such as LSD need only be taken once before a person is so sensitized to it that they can re-create the experience even while sober. The result is a permanently expanded consciousness.

TIMOTHY LEARY (1920–1996)

◎ The son of President Eisenhower's dentist and psychology lecturer at Harvard University took LSD at least once a week in 1966. When it was banned the following year, Leary contested the illegalization of LSD as well as cannabis illegalization in court, citing freedom of religion. He associated the idea of inner freedom through LSD with sexual liberation—"The Politics of Eroticism." *"Listen! Wake up! You are God!"* At their peak, Leary's Brotherhood of Eternal Love smuggled several million dollars' worth of cannabis into the United States every week. Leary was arrested in 1970, but the terrorist organization the Weather Underground broke him out of prison and helped him escape to Algeria. In 1972, the CIA caught up with *"the most dangerous man in America"* (President Nixon) in Afghanistan and sentenced him to fifteen years in prison, but Leary was released in 1976 after agreeing to testify against his former comrades.

KEN KESEY (1935–2001)

◎ With the money he earned from his 1960 novel, *One Flew Over the Cuckoo's Nest*, Kesey bought La Honda, a ranch fifty miles south of San Francisco, where he sponsored the so-called Acid Tests. Anyone who wanted to participate had to dress as outlandishly as possible and for a $1 cover charge could drink as much of the orange Kool-Aid and LSD mixture as they wanted. Music was usually courtesy of the Warlocks, the band later known as the Grateful Dead. A group of permanent La Honda residents, including poets, musicians, and hedonists, became the Merry Pranksters, who in 1964 took an LSD cross-country road trip in a Day-Glo-painted school bus. Tom Wolfe's book *The Electric Kool-Aid Acid Test* describes the self-destructive madness of the journey.

ALEXANDER SHULGIN (BORN 1925)

◎ The American chemist stumbled upon MDMA in 1967 and was the first to explore its euphoria-inducing effects. In the years that followed, Shulgin discovered another two hundred psychoactive substances and tested their effects with his wife, Ann, and friends. One hundred seventy-nine of the drugs were described in the appendix to Alexander and Ann's 1991 autobiography, *PIHKAL (Phenethylamines I Have Known and Loved)*—among them 2C-B, which is said to enhance sensory perception without distorting it.

TERENCE MCKENNA (1946–2000)

◎ The Canadian philosopher recommended taking large doses of hallucinogens alone if possible, in the dark and without music or other forms of outside stimulation. He believed this was the only way for people to realize their full potential. In his book *Food of the Gods* (1992), McKenna asserts that early man's ability to evolve from the apes stems from his partaking of the psilocybin-containing mushroom *Stropharia cubensis*. Five million years ago, "magic mushroom" consumption freed primates from the daily grind of survival and awakened their creative potential, resulting in both the development of language and religion and the invention of practical tools. At the same time, psychoactive mushrooms increased sexual desire and thereby increased the birth rate. Unfortunately, a climate change caused the mushrooms to disappear ten thousand years ago, and the baleful period of animal husbandry, male domination, and monotheism began.

DANIEL PINCHBECK (BORN 1966)

◎ The New York son of an abstract painter and a Beat authoress took to visiting shamans in Peru, Mexico, and Gabon. Today he is part of the self-dubbed New Edge psychedelic movement. Pinchbeck preaches above all the use of the plant-derived hallucinogen ayahuasca: *"Drugs like ayahuasca are like interfaces that allow us to take messages from other realities instead of being overwhelmed or short-circuited by them,"* and *"The thought came to me that human consciousness is like a flower that blossoms from the earth. The stem and the roots are invisible cords, etheric filaments that lead back to a greater, extradimensional being. Our separation from that larger being was only a temporary illusion."*

Like many esoterics, Pinchbeck believes that December 21, 2012, the last day of the five-thousand-year Mayan calendar cycle, will mean the end of the known world. The Aztec deity Quetzalcoatl—a feathered serpent—delivered him the message that he is a prophet. Only a psychedelic awakening could avert catastrophe and convey mankind to a new, nonlinear time.

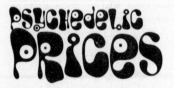

The amount of money that the author Daniel Pinchbeck paid for the drugs he used in his book *Breaking Open the Head*:

IBOGA: $600
Pinchbeck met shaman Tsanga Jean Moutamba (who calls himself "King") twenty-five miles outside of Lambaréné in Gabon. King gave him a long shopping list (red parrot feathers, one mirror, cassis liqueur, etc.) and wanted to renegotiate the price shortly before the ingestion ceremony.

AYAHUASCA: $2,000
The American tour company Sentient Experimentals charges around $2,000 for a trip to the Sequoia Indian territory in the rainforests of Ecuador. It was there that Pinchbeck tried the hallucinogenic ayahuasca, or yagé, drink.

DPT: <u>$125</u>
Ordered from a mail-order catalogue
to his home in New York. The yellow
powder, which is closely related to the
natural hallucinogen DMT, put Pinchbeck into parallel worlds of shattering
clarity. For weeks the author thought
that his apartment was possessed: A mirror falls off the wall, a mysterious insect
sits in a drawer, the rooms seem electri-
cally charged. Meditation and a friend's
Mexican exorcism set make it possible for
him to return to reality. His conclusion:
*"I strongly suspect an ordinary death is
not the worst thing that can happen to*

*a human being. There may be far worse
fates."*

PSILOCYBIN MUSHROOMS: <u>$70</u>
Pinchbeck and his girlfriend Laura
attended a Mazatec Indian sacred
mushroom ceremony in Huautla de
Jimenez, Mexico. Standing before an
altar decorated with Christian symbols
(holy virgin, the cross), the shaman
distributed a brew with ten fluorescent
green mushrooms. Pinchbeck himself
experienced only sharpened perception,
but another participant wept and begged
God for forgiveness.

THE GREATEST
REVELATIONS OF LSD PRIEST

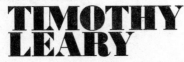

TIMOTHY LEARY

> **❝** *Yes, I listen to the trees and hear what they say and I
> think that they hear what I say. Not what I say, since
> trees don't speak English, but the trees are very aware of what I'm
> doing to them and to the ground around them. And by me I
> don't mean Timothy Leary. They don't talk that language.* **❞**

> **❝** *It's my ambition to be the holiest, wisest, most beneficial
> man alive today. Now this may sound megalomanic,
> but I don't see why. I don't see why every person
> who lives in the world shouldn't have that ambition.* **❞**

> **❝** *LSD is a specific cure for homosexuality. (. . .) We've had many cases of
> long-term homosexuals who, under LSD, discover that they are not only
> genitally but genetically male, but that they are basically attracted to females. The
> most famous and public example of such cases is that of Allen Ginsberg, who has
> openly stated that the first time he turned on to women was during an
> LSD session several years ago. But this is only one of many such cases.* **❞**

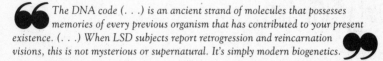

> *I don't intend to send my future children to schools. I'd rather have them take heroin than go to a first-grade grammar school in this country.*

> *The DNA code (. . .) is an ancient strand of molecules that possesses memories of every previous organism that has contributed to your present existence. (. . .) When LSD subjects report retrogression and reincarnation visions, this is not mysterious or supernatural. It's simply modern biogenetics.*

> *In general, I predict that psychedelic drugs will be used in schools in the very near future as educational devices—not only drugs like marijuana and LSD, to teach kids how to use their sense organs and their cellular equipment effectively, but new and more powerful psychochemicals like RNA and other proteins which are really going to revolutionize our concepts of ourselves and educations. So that the notion about writing an essay in the first grade on your trip is not just science fiction, it's definitely going to happen.*

> *In a carefully prepared, loving LSD session, a woman can have several hundred orgasms.*

[As to how many orgasms a man can have, Leary doesn't say.]

MDMA DISCOVERER

ALEXANDER SHULGIN'S

RULES FOR PARTICIPATING IN HIS DRUG EXPERIMENTS

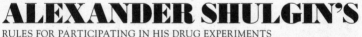

- ▶▶ Drug abstinence is required for a minimum of three days before the experiment.
- ▶▶ Each participant must bring his or her own food, beverages, and a sleeping bag for overnight stays.
- ▶▶ Ample space is provided to allow each individual to separate themselves from the group.
- ▶▶ A garden is provided to allow participants to spend time with plants and in the fresh air.
- ▶▶ Should a participant raise his or her hand, it is a signal that he or she has a reality-based concern. If a participant says, for example, "I smell smoke," it is a sign that he is genuinely troubled by the smell of smoke.
- ▶▶ Each person has veto power for any decision that affects everyone—choice of music, for example.
- ▶▶ Sexual relations between persons not in a romantic relationship are to be avoided.
- ▶▶ Couples who wish to have sex must find a private space to do so.
- ▶▶ All forms of physical violence are to be avoided. Sexual and violent fantasies may, however, be expressed and discussed.

FIVE COVETED

MARIJUANA DELICACIES

The two major marijuana strains are *Sativa* from Central Asia and *Indica* from Afghanistan. Today there are about seven hundred different varieties, with new ones bred every day. Big cannabis breeders are world stars in the stoner scene and walk the green carpet at the Stony Awards in New York.

MATANUSKA TUNDRA (ALSO: M. THUNDER)
The legendary strain from northern Alaska produces very full, large buds and lots of resin. Smells chocolatey and has a slow effect, like hiking on a majestic mountaintop. It is, however, extremely strong: *"Packs more power than an ice pack polar bear,"* as the Alaskans say.

HAZE
Though the leaves do have a violet sheen, the Jimi Hendrix song "Purple Haze" actually refers to a science fiction novel by Philip José Farmer. Haze was first cultivated in California, is a strain of sativa, and traces its genotype over four continents. The bloom time is very long (one hundred days) and the harvest small, so the variety hardly ever hits the market—and fetches record prices when it does. Haze is the champagne of grass strains, and the effect is an intense high: hallucinogenic, gentle, beguiling in new dimensions.

NORTHERN LIGHTS
One of the most famous cannabis strains, developed in Seattle in the late seventies and a Cannabis Festival favorite for years. The plant is easy to handle and grows to full size indoors in six weeks, making it extremely popular with homegrowers. Very potent, with a good "sativa high" or an invigorating, energizing buzz. It's often hallucinogenic and good for joints smoked during the day. Also very popular as a pain reliever.

ED ROSENTHAL SUPER BUD
New hybrid cross of the *Indica* and *Sativa* varieties. Breeder Ben Dronkers writes, *"Buds that swell upwards and outwards to crazy sizes. A strong and incredibly sweet aroma of pineapple-punch."* The gourmet strain was developed over several decades in Holland and named after Ed Rosenthal, the California gardener and guru to all cannabis breeders.

BIG BUDDHA CHEESE
The new sort triumphed at the 2006 Cannabis Cup in Amsterdam. Breeder Big Buddha came onstage and received a grand standing ovation from the usually rather serene hemp friends. Cheese is a variant of the English skunk; both bear the name because of their distinctive smell. Big Buddha's version is potent but without overpowering undertones.

EXCEPTIONAL THERAPY METHODS

NARCONON
✳ A drug treatment organization with close ties to the Church of Scientology. Long trips to the sauna are supposed to cleanse the body, long-winded conversations to clear the head. Christiane F. reports how her drug therapy began by touching one wall, then the other, for hours on end.

NEURO-ELECTRIC THERAPY
✳ Also called the Black Box. Electroacupuncture: Electrical current is applied to acupuncture needles. It is supposed to lessen withdrawal symptoms.

BLOOD TRANSFUSION
✳ In his heroin-addicted heyday, Rolling Stone Keith Richards was rumored to have undergone regular blood transfusions in Switzerland. This would entail either a dialysis-like treatment (useless, since drugs leave the bloodstream fairly quickly) or a kind of blood oxygen enrichment (laughable, because it's expensive and probably doesn't work). What makes this therapy stand out from the rest: The patient isn't trying to kick the habit, just get the body in better shape to keep up the addiction.

NARCOTIC SLEEP
✳ Sounds like a dream come true: The heroin addict is injected with a general anaesthetic and wakes up "clean" afterward. This therapy is controversial, though. For one, it only provides relief for physical symptoms and does nothing for the addiction. Also, a comparative study at the University at Buffalo observed worrisome side effects (pneumonia, bipolar disorders). Plus, it's expensive.

SYNANON
✳ Self-help group for drug addicts, founded in 1958 by Chuck Dederich in Santa Monica, California. The group uses no replacement drugs such as methadone. Critics attacked the organization's totalitarian power structure. All contact to the outside world, even to parents and relatives, is prohibited during the first six months.

SOBER CHIP
✳ The actress Lindsay Lohan has occasionally been spotted wearing an Alcoholics Anonymous chip printed with the words "90 days" as an expression of her three-month sobriety. Standard issue for AA members, but also the perfect way to attract attention.

FRIEND NUMBER 9

Diego Armando Maradona

"It was the hand of God," the Argentine soccer player explained after shooting a goal with his fist in the June 22, 1986, World Cup quarterfinal against England. Three months prior he had been invited by the Neapolitan Camorra, who ruled the local drug trade, to a party as their guest of honor. A fateful meeting for Diego Armando Maradona (born 1960). He had been given steroids as a boy to make him grow, and later was treated with cortisone shots to keep him in the game despite injuries, but the athlete discovered cocaine while playing for Barcelona and brought his habit to full bloom in Naples. In 1991 his urine tested positive for cocaine, and he was locked up for fifteen months and sentenced to an additional fourteen months on probation. Three years later, Maradona fired an air rifle at journalists gathered outside his home and injured five people. That same year he tested positive for the stimulant ephedrine and was incarcerated for another fifteen months. After a cocaine overdose in 2000, Maradona was admitted to a clinic in Buenos Aires and began a recovery program at his friend Fidel Castro's home in Cuba. Irritated neighbors of the ex-soccer player complained of his nightly firework displays and mask of Al Qaeda leader Osama bin Laden. His Colombian "diet consultant" was arrested in 2003 with two kilos of cocaine. Maradona had his stomach stapled in 2004 and lost 110 pounds.

Safer Sniffing

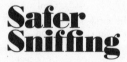

Snorting cocaine, ketamine, speed, and heroin with a rolled-up bill or drinking straw is very common but can cause infections (herpes, hepatitis). This can be avoided by sticking to the following rules of thumb:

CHOP THE DRUGS VERY FINE
—The finer the powder, the less likely that crystals will injure nasal membranes.

USE YOUR OWN TOOTER—Doing so prevents infection. If you don't happen to have anything handy, be the first to use or at least roll it the other way.

CAREFUL WITH THE CUT STRAWS
—They're sharper than they look.

NO DOLLAR BILLS—Bank notes are always dirty; try using a rolled-up Post-it note instead.

MEMORABLE

Drug Deaths

✚ JOHN BELUSHI

The actor well known for his hell-raising lifestyle spent his last night with Robin Williams and Robert De Niro, then with a groupie called Cathy Smith. She injected him with a "speedball" (a mixture of heroin and cocaine). Belushi was found dead on the morning of March 5, 1982, in his hotel room at the Chateau Marmont in Los Angeles. Smith was sentenced to eighteen months in prison for manslaughter.

✚ JOHN BONHAM

The Led Zeppelin drummer choked on his own vomit on October 25, 1980, at the home of guitarist Jimmy Page. Blood tests showed no other drugs besides alcohol. At that time, Page also owned an occult bookstore in London and had moved into the late Satanist and drug expert Aleister Crowley's (*Diary of a Drug Fiend*) rural estate.

✚ TRUMAN CAPOTE

Alcohol, pills, and cocaine caused hallucinations in his final years; his brain also showed measurable shrinkage. The author died on August 25, 1984, of liver cirrhosis, phlebitis, and multiple drug intoxication.

✚ NICK DRAKE

The musician died on November 25, 1974, of an overdose of the antidepressant Tryptizol. His parents heard him get up in the night and eat a bowl of cornflakes. The first thing his mother saw when she came to wake him the next day were *"his long, long legs."*

✚ FALCO

He wanted to die like James Dean, the Austrian singer ("Rock Me Amadeus") once said. In 1996 Falco (legal name Johann Hölzel) took up residence in the Dominican Republic, where he perished in a car accident on February 6, 1998. According to autopsy reports, Falco's blood contained traces of alcohol and cocaine. The music video and foreboding mood characterizing his last single, "Out of the Dark (Into the Light)," quickly led to speculation that the fatal accident was in fact a suicide. Little supporting evidence can confirm the theory.

✚ RAINER WERNER FASSBINDER

In 1980 the legendary German director wanted to film Pitigrilli's novel *Cocaine*, "a *film to tell something about the drug, about its effects, and about a person with the power to decide either for or against drugs, fully aware that the decision to take drugs shortens life, also but makes it more intense."*

Autopsy blood tests following his death on June 10, 1982, traced positive amounts of both barbiturates and cocaine.

✚ JERRY GARCIA

The Grateful Dead founder was a longtime cocaine and heroin addict; he suffered a heart attack and died on August 9, 1995, at the Serenity Knolls drug rehabilitation center in Forest Knolls, California. The ice cream manufacturer *Ben & Jerry's* used black cherries for Cherry Garcia, the flavor named after Garcia, in the weeks following his death.

✚ JUDY GARLAND

The chubby child star took appetite suppressants and sleeping pills on MGM Film Studios' recommendation. Later she became addicted to pills and alcohol. The forty-seven-year-old overdosed on Seconal and died on June 22, 1969.

✚ BILLIE HOLIDAY

The alcoholic singer smoked opium until it damaged her vocal cords. She then switched to heroin. Singer Anita O'Day wrote of Holiday: *"I wasn't only in awe of her singing. I was in awe of her habit. She didn't cook up on a spoon. Man, she used a small tunafish can and shot 10 cc into her feet. (Later, I understand she ran out of veins all over her body. So she used those on each side of her vagina. One sure thing, no narc was going to bust her for fresh tracks.)"*

Holiday died of heart failure and liver cirrhosis on July 17, 1959. She had taken heroin even while being in the hospital. O'Day also died of an overdose on March 4, 1966.

✚ HOWARD HUGHES

The pilot, airplane developer, film producer, and entrepreneur spent the latter part of the 1950s secluded in darkened hotel rooms, ate almost nothing but ice cream, collected his urine in milk bottles, and rarely cut his hair or fingernails. Addicted to codeine and Valium, he died on April 5, 1976, in an airplane over Texas. The official cause of death was kidney failure. His blood also contained 1.7 micrograms of codeine, usually considered a fatal dose. Hughes weighed only 99 pounds at the time of his death and X-rays showed hypodermic needles still stuck inside of his arm. The FBI could only identify him with fingerprints.

✚ HAROLD HUNTER

The professional skateboarder and actor (*Kids*) was discovered dead on the afternoon of February 17, 2006, in his Lower East Side apartment. Cocaine was found both in and near his body.

✚ RUSSELL JONES—AKA OL' DIRTY BASTARD
After a glorious career as one of hip-hop's most innovative stars and a notorious series of legal problems (robbery, shootings, failure to pay support for some of his thirteen children), Jones collapsed in the New York recording studio of his band Wu-Tang Clan on November 13, 2004. He died of the combination of prescription painkiller Tramadol and the high amounts of cocaine in his body.

✚ MARILYN MONROE
Housekeeper Eunice Murray discovered Monroe, who had been addicted to pills for a number of years, dead on August 5, 1962. The cause of death was deemed an overdose of the barbiturate Nembutal. A popular conspiracy theory alleges that the Kennedy clan was behind the presumed suicide.

✚ KEITH MOON
The Who drummer appeared in the musical *Tommy* as Uncle Ernie, a pedophile who masturbates to sweaty lingerie and abuses his nephew. Moon died on September 7, 1978, from an overdose of Heminevrin, a drug prescribed to treat his alcoholism.

✚ MARCO PANTANI
The cyclist and winner of the Tour de France and Giro d'Italia was found dead in his hotel room in Rimini on February 14, 2004. He died of a heart failure due to cocaine overdose.

✚ RIVER PHOENIX
Declared dead on October 31, 1993, at Cedars-Sinai Medical Center in Los Angeles. The actor died of a "speedball" evidently taken at the Viper Room nightclub. The vegan's blood also showed traces of cough suppressants and cannabis.

✚ ELVIS PRESLEY
Found dead on August 16, 1977, on the floor of his bathroom. It is said that he died while sitting on the toilet—wearing reading glasses—perusing a book on the Shroud of Turin. Presley was addicted to Mandrax, Valium, Ritalin, codeine, and diverse barbiturates, all the work of Dr. George "Nick" Nichopoulos, who prescribed the singer a total of five thousand pills in the last seven months of his life.

✚ JEAN SEBERG
The actress famous for her role in Godard's film *Breathless* actively supported the Black Panther Party. In her seventh month of pregnancy, FBI director J. Edgar Hoover circulated rumors that child was not fathered by her husband, Romain Gary, but by a black activist. The distress caused Seberg to suffer a premature labor and the child was stillborn. She became severely depressed, developed an addiction to pills and alcohol, and made several attempts to end her life, including throwing herself under a Paris subway.

She survived, but Seberg was discovered dead on September 8, 1979, in a Paris suburb, lying in the backseat of her parked car with large amounts of alcohol and barbiturates in her blood. In her hand was a suicide note: *"Forgive me. I can no longer live with my nerves."* It is unclear how she—without glasses and high as a kite—managed to drive herself to the 16th Arrondissement.

✚ EDIE SEDGWICK

The girl from a prestigious family embodied both the thrills and hazards of 1960s bohemia. She worked as a model before meeting Andy Warhol, who made her the "queen of the Factory." Sedgwick used speed and LSD, starred in a few of Warhol's films, and associated with Bob Dylan's clan, where she took even more drugs and was later dropped. The socialite was found lying dead next to husband Michael Post on the morning of November 16, 1971, having overdosed on barbiturates. In the movie *Ciao! Manhattan*, Sedgwick says: *"I thought drugs were like strawberries and peaches. Strange, zombie-like . . . Speed is the ultimate, all-time high."*

✚ DON SIMPSON

Died of a heart attack in his bathroom on January 19, 1996. His biographer, Charles Fleming, maintains that the film producer spent $60,000 every month on drugs. At the moment of his death, Simpson was reportedly reading—with reading glasses—a book about Oliver Stone.

✚ ANNA NICOLE SMITH

After lurid speculations about the fatherhood, the wannabe-heiress of a billion-dollar fortune gave birth to her daughter Dannielynn on September 7, 2006. She had apparently been taking methadone until the eighth month of pregnancy. Her twenty-year-old son, Daniel, died during a visit to the hospital from a combination of Zoloft, Lexapro, and methadone. On February 8, 2007, Smith's body was found at the Seminole Hard Rock Hotel in Hollywood, Florida. She had taken a lethal dose of chloral hydrate, a powerful sedative, along with seven other prescription drugs (Valium, Benadryl, Klonopin, Nordiazepam, Temezepam, Oxazepam, Lorazepam).

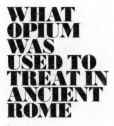

WHAT OPIUM WAS USED TO TREAT IN ANCIENT ROME

Insomnia
Shortness of breath
Elephantitis
Epilepsy
Scorpion stings
Snake bites
Pestilence
Restlessness
Coughing
Fever
Melancholy
Colic
Vomiting blood
Aphonia
Vertigo
Deafness
Stroke
Jaundice
Leprosy
Abdominal cramps
Infections of the uterus

✚ SID VICIOUS

The former Sex Pistols bass player awoke in his bed at the New York Chelsea Hotel on October 2, 1978, to find his girlfriend Nancy Spungen in the bathroom, killed by a knife wound to the stomach. Vicious, who, like Spungen, was a heroin addict, immediately left the hotel in search of methadone. Some time later he placed a call for help. His reports to police were muddled. When asked why he left his girlfriend in the hotel, he answered, "Oh, I am a dog." Vicious was released on $50,000 bail and died of a heroin overdose at his homecoming party on February 2, 1979.

✚ DINAH WASHINGTON

The singer took amphetamine diet pills in a desperate attempt to lose weight before an appearance. Combining them with alcohol and barbiturates cost her her life on December 14, 1963.

✚ TENNESSEE WILLIAMS

The playwright (A Streetcar Named Desire) choked on the cap of a nasal spray bottle that had fallen into his mouth during use. His inability to cough it out could have been a result of his drug- and alcohol-impaired reflexes.

✚ PAULA YATES

After waking from an overdose of Valium and Bailey's, the British television presenter said, "Good God, I almost pulled a Marilyn Monroe." She lost custody of her three daughters from ex-husband Bob Geldof after an opium stash was found in a candy bag under her bed. Her new lover, INXS singer Michael Hutchence, had apparently introduced her to the substance. His suicide caused her to fall into a deep depression. Yates did not reawaken on Sunday, September 17, 2000, after choking on her own vomit with heroin, vodka, and medication in her blood.

STORE-BOUGHT DRUGS AND HOW THEY WORK

AFTERSHAVE

✖ The cheap, readily available liquid is 97% pure alcohol, twice as strong as commercially available vodka.

ETHER

✖ The narcotic ether only inhibits the cerebrum—though unlike opium it also compromises involuntary regions such as the reparatory center. Its effects are similar to alcohol in their reduction of self-criticism, an effect that can lead to increased arousal and euphoria. People began to drink ether instead of spirits in mid-nineteenth-century Ireland because of the high alcohol taxes; some pastors began to recommend ether as an alcohol replacement. The heavy ether fumes made it hard to breathe in pubs. Addicts can increase their dose to up to

100 grams daily—a deadly dose for ether first-timers. French writers Maupassant and Baudelaire used ether to battle the anxiety caused by syphilis infections. Maupassant said, *"It seemed to me that I had tasted of the Tree of Knowledge."*

BUTANE

✖ Inhaled from cigarette lighters, usually mixed with the chemically related substance propane. Dangerous due to a lowered oxygen intake and risk of fire.

COFFEE

✖ The caffeine contained in coffee beans is a purine alkaloid and one of the oldest, most easily digested stimulants in the world. One cup of coffee contains between 50 and 100 milligrams of the substance. Sufis and dervishes have used the stimulant to pursue religious rituals for nights on end. In East Africa, the coffee bean is attributed divine powers.

NUTMEG

✖ The spice contains safrole and myristicin, which are closely related to MDC or MDMA (ecstasy). One matchbox-full of ground nutmeg is enough for a substantial high, though the toxicant also causes nausea. The jazz musician Charlie Parker took it on a regular basis.

CONTACT ADHESIVE

✖ Glue sniffers call it huffing: The adhesive is squeezed into a plastic baggie to prevent the fumes from escaping, then inhaled directly from the bag. The high is short and intense, with a relaxing, euphoric effect caused by the organic solvents, including toluene, hexane, and hydrocarbons. The long-term effects are disastrous, and because of its affordability and accessibility the drug is used all over the world. Other inhalants include rubber cement, nail polish, nail polish remover, benzene, defroster, stain remover, fire extinguishing fluid, and paint thinner.

LAUGHING GAS

✖ *"My God! I knew everything!"* said the writer Oscar Wilde of laughing gas's effects. Laughing gas is widely available in hardware stores and auto shops. Cool Whip brand whipped cream cartridges and other aerosol-pumped foods also contain up to 100% laughing gas as a propellant (nitrous oxide, N_2O, also known as a food additive with the designation E942). The cartridge contents are typically emptied into a balloon for better dosing, and the sweet-smelling gas has a strong pain-killing, slightly narcotic effect when inhaled. Effects can be felt in a concentration of 20% in the breathed air. A laughing gas high is short, passing after only five minutes.

RED BULL

✖ The decade's most successful new soft drink and founding member of the energy drink product group. Active ingredients in the beverage include caffeine, sugar, vitamins, and the ominous taurine, an organic acid with an amino group that is produced by the human body but can also be extracted from bulls. Most taurine is synthetically produced. The performance-enhancing effects promised in Red Bull ads have yet to be proved.

VITAMIN B$_{12}$ (1000 MCG)

✖ The vitamin B$_{12}$ is crucial to neurotransmitter brain activity. The effect is perceived as a slight boost in mental fitness. The white or pink pills can also be crushed and snorted, though they do have a vaguely meaty smell.

NYQUIL

✖ A combination of the active ingredients dextromethorphan, paracetamol, ephedrine, and doxylamine, commonly used to treat nighttime cold and influenza symptoms. Dextromethorphan (DXM) is a morphium-related cough suppressant, and ephedrine counts among the many sympathomimetic drugs with adrenalinelike effects. The antihistamine doxylamine, on the other hand, acts as a tranquilizer. Some ladies in nursing homes have their young community service volunteers bring them one to two bottles daily, and stay high on the substance for hours on end. Eminem also loves NyQuil: "*I had too much NyQuil and Vivarin again. Lost my stomach all over the place.*"

THE DUMBEST DRUG MOVIES

REEFER MADNESS (1936)

✤ The anti-cannabis film shows an old man heedlessly run over, coltish dancing at a private party, lewd women, and an ensuing rape. A court trial and sentencing follows in the second half, dragged out in mind-numbing detail. Actually the cannabis users just seem drunk the whole time.

TOMMY (1975)

✤ Filming the Who's *Tommy* rock opera was the zenith of weird British director Ken Russell's short-lived success. Tommy can neither see nor hear after witnessing his stepfather murder his father, a World War II captain unexpectedly returned home. One day the Acid Queen, played by Tina Turner, leads him into the attic. Initially clad in blood-red platforms and a blood-red cloak, she mutates into a steely suit of armor pinned with dozens of syringes. The armor opens and Tommy steps inside and is transformed into his dead father, Jesus on the cross, and a snake-infested skeleton. The Acid Queen's healing is a failure. Instead Tommy, who is still blind and deaf, becomes a pinball virtuoso. He performs in a giant arena and Elton John, decked out in yard-high shoes and oversized glasses, sings of his wondrous art. In the meantime Tommy's mother proceeds to squander her famous son's income in a white luxury suite, though she eventually succumbs to guilt and is buried by baked beans that come sloshing out of the television.

CHEECH AND CHONG: UP IN SMOKE (1978)

✤ Comedians Tommy Chong and Cheech Marin essentially pioneered the stoner movie with their six-part series, *Cheech and Chong*. In *Up in Smoke*, the two agree to drive a van from Mexico into the United States, unaware that it is made completely of hashish. Of course the van is set aflame in the grand finale, cheering even the police.

PULP FICTION (1994)

✤ Though director Quentin Tarantino's film managed to revive the suit and tie, we can't say he did the same for heroin. Uma Thurman gets an adrenaline shot rammed in her heart after an overdose, and John Travolta, who still manages to look rather casual even after the first fix, is later shot while sitting on the toilet.

TRAINSPOTTING (1996)

✤ Apparently director Danny Boyle wanted his film to look neo-expressionistic, surrealistic, and grimy at the same time—and so the movie dated itself even faster than the Irvine Welsh novel from which it was adapted. Noticeable is Boyle's fondness for fecal humor: Ewan McGregor disappears in the Worst Toilet in Scotland to retrieve the opium suppositories that he had carelessly slipped into his behind. The soundtrack is all too predictable: Greatest hits from the likes of drug friends Iggy Pop, Lou Reed, and Underworld.

FEAR AND LOATHING IN LAS VEGAS (1998)

✤ Somehow Monty Python's Terry Gilliam managed to persuade actor Johnny Depp to play a role where for once he wouldn't look cute. As Hunter S. Thompson, Depp is seen in a very unflattering jacket, half bald and waddling around like a long-legged duck. The film is about the creator and only practicer of Gonzo journalism, the roving reporter who traveled around with a suitcase full of cocaine, mescaline, and LSD, accompanied by lawyer/agent/buddy the Samoan Dr. Gonzo (Benicio del Toro). In a flashback we see Thompson in a club restroom taking his first hit of liquid LSD: He pours half of it in his mouth; the other half lands on his lumberjack shirt and is sucked out by a hippie. It only gets worse from there, until Thompson thinks he's sitting in a bar full of giant reptiles.

SPUN (2002)

✤ Overexcited crystal meth movie by Swedish music director Jonas Åkerlund (*Ray of Light*), rife with broken teeth, paranoia, dilapidation, strip bars, and sex shops. A small-time dealer played by actor John Leguizamo dons absurdly low-riding leather pants; later in the movie he appears wearing only a jack-off sock. A pimply customer stares at a gorilla giving himself a fix in the Insane Clown Posse video game Juggalo Championshit Wrestling and starting to masturbate (the gorilla, not the customer). Mickey Rourke attempts a comeback in his role as a drug cooker in cowboy boots. The film works with rapid-fire montage to create a kind of silent film effect. Hard, electronic noises signal the moment when the speed reaches the brain. Most famous scene: Ross (Jason Schwartzman) has ferocious, neverending sex—defused by visual blur and animation—with a stripper and leaves her, mouth taped and handcuffed on the bed, for later.

STONED (2005)

❧ Judging from this movie, the last days of musician Brian Jones's life must have been rather dull. Down at Cotchford Farm, the former home of writer A. A. Milne (*Winnie the Pooh*), the asthmatic addict sought comfort in alcohol, hashish, and sadism against women and employees after falling out with the other Rolling Stones. A flashback sequence shows Jones with then-girlfriend Anita Pallenberg on the set of Volker Schlöndorff's *A Degree of Murder*—surreal and with a little whip sex. This must be how a seventies *Playboy* editor imagined an LSD trip.

ANIMALS AND THEIR NATURAL INTOXICANTS

YELLOW MEADOW ANTS—SECRE-TIONS OF THE LOMECHUSA BEETLE

❧ The worker ants take the beetle and nourish it. Excessive consumption of the beetles' secretions leads to an inability to work, and queens become incapable of reproduction.

CATS—CATNIP

❧ Catnip contains nepeta, which simulates a tomcat's mating scent. Many cats experience an erection from catnip; female cats will assume a breeding position.

LLAMAS—COCA LEAVES

❧ Human coca consumption probably began when llamas were first domesticated around 5000 B.C. Crossing the Andean highlands, the animals had to do without their usual sources of food and ate coca leaves instead. Not only do the leaves contain the stimulant cocaine, they are also extremely nutritious. A

quantity of 100 grams contains 42.6 grams of carbohydrate, 18.6 grams of protein, as well as calcium, iron, phosphorous, riboflavin, and vitamins A and E.

PIGS—TRUFFLES

❧ Truffles contain the steroid androstenol, which is produced in the boor's testicles during courtship. The hormone makes boors more aggressive and sows more willing to mate. Androstenol can also be found in men's underarm perspiration.

PIGS—IBOGA ROOTS

❧ Pigs eagerly dig for the hallucinogenic root and jump around wildly after eating it.

THRUSH—HAWTHORN BERRIES

❧ The birds greedily descend on the saponin-containing berries, then flutter through the air tipsy and often smack into windshields.

FRIEND NUMBER 10
Steve Jobs

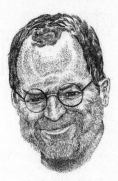

A teenaged Steve Jobs (born 1955) thought he'd died
and gone to heaven when he landed his first summer job at Hewlett Packard. He was a loner and an
absolute tech nerd; now he was allowed to tight-
en screws at California's most illustrious tech
corporation. As originally reported by Jeffrey
S. Young and William L. Simon in *iCon*, when
asked by colleagues to name the best thing in
the world, *"Electronics!"* was his enthusiastic
reply. His foreman's answer was *"fucking."*

   "I learned a lot that summer," Jobs recalled later. *"I got
stoned for the first time; I discovered Shakespeare, Dylan Thomas,
and all that classic stuff. I read* Moby Dick *and took creative writing class-
es."* Pot-smoking tinkerers like Jobs were called "wireheads" in the sixties—
they were cooler than regular nerds who had only electronic parts on their minds.

At sixteen, he sported shoulder-length hair and appeared less and less at school.
Afternoons were spent with his then-girlfriend Chris-Ann Brennan; the two
took long walks, drank wine, smoked pot, and felt a deep, spiritual bond in
their mutual rejection of authority. Wanting to take an LSD trip together,
they retreated into a wheat field. *"All of a sudden the wheat field was
playing Bach,"* he recalled. *"It was the most wonderful experience of
my life up to that point. I felt like the conductor of this symphony
with Bach coming through the wheat field."*

Soon after that he dropped out of college and was
hired by Atari, but then he traveled to the Himalayas to
expand his consciousness with Far Eastern mysticism.
Jobs found a guru, shaved his head, and returned
to California in an orange-colored toga, where the
nineteen-year-old returned to his job at Atari. In 1976,
two years later, he and partner Steve Wozniak brought
the world's first personal computer onto the market for $666.
The models Apple 1 and Apple 2 marked the beginning of Apple
Incorporated, quickly developing the Zen disciple's taste for another
intoxicant. "When I was twenty-three, I had a net worth of a million dollars. At twenty-four, it was over ten million dollars. At twenty-five, it was over a
hundred million," Jobs has often been quoted as saying. In addition to Apple and Mac
computers, his iPod was also a world success. Jobs is currently worth $3.3 billion; selling
his animation studio Pixar made him the largest individual stockholder at Disney.

Tramadol

Tramadol is the only opium derivative that is not considered a controlled substance in many countries, including the United States and Canada. It is a white, crystalline, bitter, and odorless powder that dissolves readily in water. The active ingredient is also sold under the following tradenames:

Adamon—Costa Rica, Dominican Republic, El Salvador, Guatemala, Honduras, Nicaragua, Panama
Analab—Thailand
Analdol—Israel
Andalpha—Indonesia
Bellatram—Indonesia
Biodalgic—France
Contramal—France, India
Contramal LP—France
Dolana—Indonesia
Dolotral—Philippines
Dromadol—England
Exopen—Korea
Katrasic—Indonesia
Mabron—China, Israel, Thailand
Mosepan—Philippines
Nonalges—Indonesia

Omnidol—Colombia
O.P. Pain—Korea
Pengesic—Singapore
Penimadol—Korea
Prontofort—Mexico
Radol—Indonesia
Sefmal—Hong Kong, Singapore
Takadol—France
Tamolan—Thailand
Tandol—Korea
Tarol—Israel
Topalgic—France
Trabar—Israel
Tradol—Mexico
Tramadex—Israel
Tramagetic—Germany
Tramagit—Germany
Tramahexal—South Africa
Tramake—England, Ireland
Tramal—Austria, Bulgaria, China, Colombia, Ecuador, Germany, Hong Kong, Israel, Malaysia, Netherlands, Peru, Philippines, Switzerland, Taiwan, Thailand
Tramal SR—Australia
Tramazac—India, South Africa
Tramed—Taiwan
Tramol—Poland

Trasedal—France
Trasik—Indonesia
TRD-Contin—India
Trexol—Mexico
Tridol—Korea
Ultram—United States
Unitral—Philippines
Urgendol—India
Zamadol—England
Zodol—Peru
Zumatran—Indonesia
Zydol—England, Ireland
Zytram BD—New Zealand
Zytram XL SR—Korea

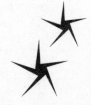

COCAINE PRICES IN THE USA

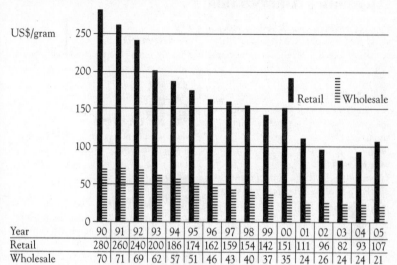

US$/gram

Retail ☰Wholesale

Year	90	91	92	93	94	95	96	97	98	99	00	01	02	03	04	05
Retail	280	260	240	200	186	174	162	159	154	142	151	111	96	82	93	107
Wholesale	70	71	69	62	57	51	46	43	40	37	35	24	26	24	24	21

HEROIN PRICES IN THE USA

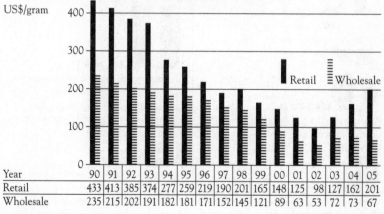

US$/gram

Retail ☰Wholesale

Year	90	91	92	93	94	95	96	97	98	99	00	01	02	03	04	05
Retail	433	413	385	374	277	259	219	190	201	165	148	125	98	127	162	201
Wholesale	235	215	202	191	182	181	171	152	145	121	89	63	53	72	73	67

Source: UN 2007 World Drug Report

THE TWELVE STEPS OF
Alcoholics Anonymous

First created by Alcoholics Anonymous, these twelve steps to recovery now form the basis for countless other drug therapies.

1st step
We admitted we were powerless over alcohol—that our lives had become unmanageable.

2nd step
Came to believe that a Power greater than ourselves could restore us to sanity.

3rd step
Made a decision to turn our will and our lives over to the care of God as we understood Him.

4th step
Made a searching and fearless moral inventory of ourselves.

5th step
Admitted to God, to ourselves, and to another human being the exact nature of our wrongs.

6th step
Were entirely ready to have God remove all these defects of character.

7th step

Humbly asked Him to remove our shortcomings.

8th step
Made a list of all persons we had harmed and became willing to make amends to them all.

9th step
Made direct amends to such people wherever possible, except when to do so would injure them or others.

10th step
Continued to take personal inventory and when we were wrong promptly admitted it.

11th step
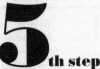
Sought through prayer and meditation to improve our conscious contact with God, as we understood Him, praying only for knowledge of His will for us and the power to carry that out.

12th step

Having had a spiritual awakening as the result of these steps, we tried to carry this message to alcoholics, and to practice these principles in all our affairs.

IMAGINARY
DRUGS FROM LITERATURE, FILM, AND TELEVISON

SOMA—ALDOUS HUXLEY, *BRAVE NEW WORLD*
❉ A thoughtless and happy-making tranquilizer, named after the historical Indian drug Soma: "*Two thousand pharmacologists and bio-chemists were subsidized in A.P. 178. Six years later it was being produced commercially. The perfect drug. Euphoric, narcotic, pleasantly hallucinant. All the advantages of Christianity and alcohol; none of their defects.*"

MOKSHA—ALDOUS HUXLEY, *ISLAND*
❉ According to Hindu belief, Moksha is the soul's release from physical life and suffering, the never-ending cycle of birth and death. In his last novel, *Island* (1962), Huxley describes a positive utopia in which the LSD and mescaline-reminiscent drug Moksha helps to expand consciousness and come to terms with dying.

MOLOKO PLUS—ANTHONY BURGESS, *A CLOCKWORK ORANGE*
❉ *Moloko* is the Russian word for milk. At the Korova milkbar, milk is spiked with either vellocet (for an extra-alert, ultra-violent effect) or synthemesc (the synthetically produced hallucinogen mescaline).

CAN-D, CHEW-Z—PHILIP K. DICK,
THE THREE STIGMATA OF PALMER ELDRITCH
❉ Life on Mars is dull and bleak; the human colonists huddle miserably in shelters. For comfort, they seek refuge in the imaginary world of Perky Pat and her friends. The drug Can-D enables them to enter the toy world as into a virtual reality. Because the action figures and their accessories are expensive, different colonists are often forced to cast themselves into a single doll at the same time, a situation that often leads to wrangles. The mysterious Palmer Eldritch produces the competing drug Chew-Z, a high that, though no longer dependent upon a miniature world to achieve its effect, is permanent. Chew-Z is marketed under the slogan "God promises eternal life. We can deliver it." The hero of the novel suspects that an otherworldly, malevolent force inhabits Palmer Eldritch, a man with steel teeth, glass eyes, and metallic eyelids.

D, MEX HIT—PHILIP K. DICK, *A SCANNER DARKLY*
❉ D is extracted from a blue flower—a reference to one of the central symbols of German Romanticism. Called *Mors ontologica*, meaning "Ontological Death," or "Death of the Knowledge of Being," the use of Substance D over an extended period causes a splitting of the user's personality into two distinct parts that have no knowledge of each other. "Mex hit" is a 50–50 mix of D and heroin.

"'D,' he said aloud to his audience, 'is for Substance D. Which is for Dumbness and Despair and Desertion, the desertion of your friends from you, you from them, everyone from everyone, isolation and loneliness and hating and suspecting each other.'

'D' he said then, 'is finally Death. Slow Death, we—' He halted. 'We, the dopers,' he said, 'call it.' His voice rasped and faltered. 'As you probably know. Slow Death. From the head on down. Well, that's it.'"

VURT—JEFF NOON, *VURT*
❋ The drug Vurt is a knockoff of Philip K. Dick's imaginary drugs Can-D and Chew-Z. The users suck on colored bird feathers that allow their dreams and myths to become reality.

ECSTACIDE, FAITH SALTS, CHRISTENDINE, BUDDHINE, ALGEBRINE, AUTHENTIUM, AMNESOL, DUETINE, AND MANY MORE—STANISLAV LEM, *THE FUTUROLOGICAL CONGRESS*
❋ The name says it all when it comes to their effects: Ecstacide induces ecstasy, faith salts lead to belief, christendine to belief in Christianity in particular, buddhine to faith in Buddhism, algebrine enhances the user's math skills. Authentium creates synthetic memories, while amnesol helps to forget it all again. Duetine splits the personality and makes it possible for a person to have a discussion with him or herself.

SNOW CRASH—NEAL STEPHENSON, *SNOW CRASH*
❋ Snow Crash is a drug and computer virus in one. A drug that replicates itself, it entered the world in biblical times with the building of the Tower of Babel.

KRYPTONITE—JOE SHUSTER/JERRY SIEGEL, *SUPERMAN*
❋ The comic book hero's legendary abilities have since 1938 resonated in the work of countless filmmakers and draftsmen augmenting the powers of the man—called Clark Kent in civilian life—to near invincibility. His only weakness is Kryptonite, a fictional element from Superman's home planet that exploded shortly after the superhero's birth. Kryptonite is typically green in color; the hero loses his powers upon contact with it, suffers pain, and teeters on the brink of death. His enemies are therefore determined to acquire Kryptonite at all costs. In the film *Superman Returns*, Lex Luthor steals the substance from a meteorite exhibition; in the comic *Batman: The Dark Knight Returns*, Batman uses a little-known, obscenely expensive procedure to create a synthetic variant.

MAGIC POTION—ALBERT UDERZO/RENÉ GOSCINNY, *ASTERIX THE GAUL*
❋ The druid Getafix's magic potion plays an important role in the French comic book series. The drinker gains supernatural physical strength and helps a small village in northern Gaul (now Normandy) defend itself against Roman invasion. The recipe for the potion is a secret that passes strictly from "druid mouth to druid ear," though the

occasional shortfall in supply has revealed the following ingredients: lobster, fresh fish, mistletoe cut with a golden sickle, rock oil (alternatively: red beetroot juice). The magic potion is not risk-free; cross-reactions can occur when drinking it in combination with other potions. After having fallen into a magic potion cauldron as a little boy, Obelix the Gaul can only ingest other potions in exceptional cases.

SPICE OR MELANGE—FRANK W. HERBERT, *DUNE*
❄ A reddish-brown powder reminiscent of cinnamon. Produced by sandworms on the planet Arrakis, the drug prolongs life, allows users to see the future, strengthens the immune system, and tints the whites of the eyes blue. Spice can also be used to produce explosives, clothing, and paper.

GLITTERSTIM, CARSUNUM, RYLL SPICES—*STAR WARS* LITERARY UNIVERSE
❄ Similarities to Frank W. Herbert's Spice are striking. Glitterstim lends the user telepathic powers but also leads to a loss of control. It is secreted by a crystalline, spiderlike being that lives in deep caves. Carsunum enhances mental and physical powers but can also cause death. Ryll has a relatively weak effect and is used recreationally by workers in their free time.

NUMBER TWELVE—NICK MCDONELL, *TWELVE*
❄ A dealer supplies rich, bored, brand-crazy Manhattan youths with Number Twelve, a snorting drug with effects similar to ecstasy: *"Jessica giggles and flows off of the toilet, her face sliding easily against the porcelain and leaving a trail of sweat."*

SPACE HONEY—*FUTURAMA*
❄ Honey produced by gigantic space bees on this TV show. *"One spoonful calms you down. Two spoonfuls help you sleep. But three spoonfuls and you'll go into a sleep so deep you'll never wake up."*

SYNTHEHOL—*STAR TREK: THE NEXT GENERATION*
❄ An alcohol substitute that intoxicates without leaving a hangover.

CHEMICAL—RAY LORIGA, *TOKYO DOESN'T LOVE US ANYMORE*
❄ In the Spanish author's first novel, the dealer protagonist travels the world peddling Chemical, a retroactive drug that erases the user's memory—a few hours, days, or weeks depending on the dose. His clientele consists mainly of rootless globetrotters and occasional serial murderers who, after committing their crimes, want to return to their regular lives with a clear conscience.

ABULINIX—BENJAMIN KUNKEL, *INDECISION*
❄ The medication is a treatment against the chronic inability to make decisions.

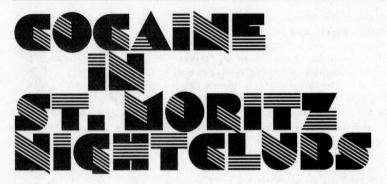

COCAINE IN ST. MORITZ NIGHTCLUBS

The Swiss resort town is as famous for its breathtaking landscape as it is for illustrious guests and their raucous parties. "Nightclub" is a loose designation in ski areas: Usually the boozing begins in so-called après-ski bars, frequently in waterproof clothing and heavy footwear.

Scientists from the Nuremberg Institute for Biomedical and Pharmaceutical Research compared drug residue traces in several gastronomic venues in St. Moritz during the 2005 ski season. The institute became known in the nineties for having discovered cocaine residue on banknotes and in the German parliament building. One of the techniques it uses is the "drug wipe" method, which consists of swiping a surface and testing the rag for the substance.

Place	Sample	Cocaine detected (in micrograms)
Diamond	Restroom, Men's, Toilet paper dispenser	98.8
	Restroom, Men's, Flush handle and toilet lid	93.3
	Restroom, Ladies', Countertop	63.1
	Restroom, Men's, Doorknob	10.6
ViVai	Restroom, Men's, Toilet paper dispenser	80.4
	Restroom, Men's, Toilet lid	49.8
	Restroom, Ladies', Countertop	30.4
	Restroom, Men's, Flush handle	19.9
	Restroom, Ladies', Soap dish	0.676
Stübli Schweizerhof	Restroom, Ladies', Countertop	13.3
	Restroom, Men's, Toilet lid	12.19
	Restroom, Ladies', Toilet lid	0.476

FRIEND NUMBER 11
Pete Doherty

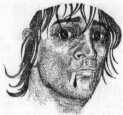

If British journalists hadn't the power to define what counts as current and important, and had supermodel Kate Moss not fallen for the romance of his self-destruction, few would have heard of the Babyshambles frontman today.

Yet not since Kurt Cobain has a rock musician been allowed to live his addictions (heroin, cocaine, crack) so publicly. In 2003, Pete Doherty (born 1979) broke into bandmate Carl Barat's flat and was subsequently sentenced to six months in prison. After that there was no shaking him from the tabloid headlines: The singer left the famed Thailand detox center Wat Tham Krabok after only three days of treatment, took methadone on an airplane to Spain, and was banned from the airline; in London he was pulled over in his Jaguar by police for speeding through the city under the heavy influence of drugs, and he told journalists that he liked to paint with the blood of his friends. Doherty's irresistible charms as a champagne junkie inspired Italian fashion designer Roberto Cavalli to book him as a model for an advertising campaign. But even before shooting to fame with his first band, the Libertines, Doherty was no stranger to relations with men. *News of the World* headlines reported that "Pete was a twenty-pound rent boy," to which the musician responded, *"There was no shame, because I kind of knew that they were just lonely pissed-up old queens. And twenty quid was a lot of money."* His relationship with Kate Moss, whom he has occasionally introduced at concerts as his fiancée, is officially over but has been so stormy that we dare not venture a prognosis: wedding, end, even deeper in the mire—anything is possible. In a brief moment of sobriety he said to *Vogue Hommes International*: *"I just don't want to go down. As Kate would say, it's not a good look."*

PRIMARY DRUG USE

AMONG PEOPLE IN THE U.S. TREATED FOR DRUG PROBLEMS		
Cannabis		46.4%
Cocaine/crack		36.7%
Amphetamines		16.2%
Opiates		15.0%
Tranquilizers		12.8%
Inhalants		7.7%
Ecstasy		0.2%

Source: UN 2007 World Drug Report   PEOPLE TREATED: 2,172,000

SPEED MUSIC

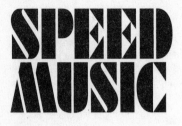

FRED ASTAIRE
🎵 Fred Astaire can be heard singing the praises of Benzedrine brand amphetamine capsules on the soundtrack to the film *You Were Never Lovelier* (1942):
"I'm like the B-19
Loaded with Benzedrine"

JERRY LEE LEWIS
🎵 The rock 'n' roll pioneer began his career performing to truckers. They threw speed pills at the nineteen-year-old onstage as a sign of their appreciation. He set his piano on fire during the Big Beat tour in 1958, the same year in which he married his thirteen-year-old cousin, Myra, and thus temporarily ended his career. The singer inadvertently shot his base player Butch Owens in the stomach on his forty-first birthday in 1976.

JOHNNY CASH
🎵 Cash developed a speed dependency while hanging around the drivers who shuttled the Grand Ole Opry stars around the country. In October 1967, after several days of neither food nor sleep, he crawled into the Nickajack Cave in Tennessee to lie down and die.

Suddenly it occurred to him that not he, but the Lord, would decide when his time had come. Cash was rehabilitated and became religious.

THE WHO
🎵 By 1961, 2.5% of all prescriptions filled by Britain's National Health Service were for amphetamine. It was the mods, though—those Vespa-driving, suit-wearing English hipsters—that popularized speed as a recreational drug. Amphetamine fueled their feeling of controlled rage; eating, drinking, and women all lost appeal. Mods are distinctive as a youth movement in that they made no music of their own but instead adopted "black music" such as R&B, soul, and Jamaican bluebeat. The Who was the first mod band to break through with songs like "I Can't Explain," "Anyway, Anyhow, Anywhere" (*"Nothing gets in my way, not even locked doors"*), and "Substitute." Their manager, Kit Lambert (also a speed addict), sent the band for a haircut and an outfitting on Carnaby Street. At concerts, the band tried to emulate their mod fans' dance steps. But the Who's trademark move was the carefully timed loss of control. Pete Townshend in particular was prone to twirling his arms

and the microphone, and regularly ended sets by smashing his guitar.

THE SMALL FACES

♣ The second most successful mod band released "Here Comes the Nice" in 1967 as the movement was pretty much over and performed it on *Top of the Pops*:
"*Here comes the nice
He knows what I need
He's always there when I need some speed.*"

BLUE CHEER

♣ Created in 1967, the Boston band named itself after an allegedly especially strong type of LSD but wound up a favorite of San Francisco tweakers and cofounder of Heavy Metal. Their six gigantic amplifiers with a total of twenty-four speakers were hellishly loud. Legend has it that a stray dog ran onstage and dropped dead.

MOTÖRHEAD

♣ *Motörhead* is American slang for speed consumption. Singer Ian "Lemmy" Kilmister founded the group in 1975 after being kicked out of space rock band Hawkwind for his heavy amphetamine habit. The LP titles *Iron Fist*, *Overkill*, and *No Sleep Till Hammersmith* speak for themselves. Motörhead's fast tempo was seminal to the heavy metal sound.

EINSTÜRZENDE NEUBAUTEN

♣ The West Berliners recorded their first single, "Für den Untergang," in 1980 under a steel highway underpass. Drummer Andrew Unruh ("*Be smart* *alright, rob the building site*") wailed on anything huge and steel: oil tanks, air shafts, massive sheet metal plates. Holes were chopped at random into their hair, clothes made out of trash and held together with screws, staples, and seatbelts, and feet were shod in stinking galoshes. Band member Alex Hacke recalled:
"*That was harder than the normal punk rockers. It was a kind of high form of ugliness. That was the most important thing for me: looking into filth (. . .) Yoghurt cups full of piss next to the bed.*"

D.A.F.

♣ In the beginning, D.A.F.— short for Deutsch-Amerikanische Freundschaft (German-American Friendship)—was a five-headed band; at the end there were only two. Because who needs guitars in the eighties? What's there to discuss? Gabi Delgado and Robert Görl were not only hard but cold. The homoerotic duo cast nary a glance in anyone else's direction; they slept in cellars, crates, or on the street. Music was only looped and played from cassettes at concerts—anticipating techno by several years— while Gabi Delgado sang his frequently fascist slogans in his very deepest voice, the most scandalous being "Dance the Mussolini, Dance the Adolf Hitler." They switched from speed to cocaine as soon as they had earned the money to do so, buying it off of Blixa Bargeld, the singer from Einstürzende Neubauten.

THE MOST DEVASTATING DRUG COMBINATIONS

KING'S MIX, CROAK: cocaine and speed

COCKTAIL, WHIZ BANG: heroin and cocaine

BACK-TO-BACK: heroin and crack

BELGIUM POT: cocaine and strychnine (cyclists' drug)

SPEEDBALL: cocaine/speed and heroin

FRISCO SPEEDBALL: cocaine and heroin and LSD

BLACK H: heroin and caffeine

BAM, BLACK BOMBER, UPS AND DOWNS: barbiturate and speed

✚ SEXSTASY: ecstasy and Viagra

CANDY FLIP: ecstasy and LSD

✚ HIPPY FLIP: ecstasy and psilo mushrooms

KITTY FLIP: ecstasy and ketamine

SPACEBASE: crack and PCP

PRODUCT IV: LSD and PCP

ZERO ZERO: hashish and opium

CRANK: amphetamine and methamphetamine

✚ FRISCO SPEED, YELLOW SUBMARINE, SUNSHINE: speed and LSD

BLUE VELVET, P.O.: antihistamine (such as pyribenzamine) and opium/codeine

✚ WHACKY STICK, SUPERGRASS: joint laced with PCP

✚ COCO PUFF, 51ER, NEVADITO, JUDY FLY: joint filled with cocaine

✚ TRIP GRASS, TRIP SHIT: marijuana and speed

✚ ATOM BOMB, THAI STICK: marijuana and heroin/opium

✚ ASTHMADOR: cigarette with stramonium and belladonna

✚ B 40: Joint with malt sugar

✚ CHRONIC, CHRON: marijuana laced with crack or cocaine

✚ TO GO ROBOTIN': smoking a joint while drinking Robitussin cough medicine

✚ JUNGLE: joint made of marijuana and hashish

✚ TURPS: oil of turpentine camphor and codeine

✚ ZNA: dill and glutamate

✚ VODKA ACID: vodka with LSD

✚ WILD GERONIMO: alcohol with barbiturates

✚ T's AND B's, B's, BOTTOMS, BETTIES: Talwin (pentazocine) and pyribenzamine

✚ PROZACCO: Prozac dissolved in Prosecco

FRIEND NUMBER 12
Mick Jagger

"We're talking heroin with the president /
Well it's a problem, sir, but it can't be bent,"
scoffed the Rolling Stones in their song "Respectable." At the time, guitarist Keith Richards
was on trial for importing narcotics to Canada. The
band never was able to hide its heartfelt connection to
substances, an image that served them well over the years.
The albums *Let It Bleed*, *Sticky Fingers*, and *Exile on Main
Street* are heavily influenced by drug use.

On February 12, 1967, Richards held a party at his home in
West Sussex. Guests included Mick Jagger, Beatle George Harrison,
art dealer Robert Fraser, and Jagger's then-girlfriend Marianne Faithfull, a descendant of Leopold Ritter von Sacher-Masoch and known by
manager Andrew Oldham as the "blond angel with tits." Canadian David
Schneidermann was also there, with plenty of Orange Sunshine, the best
LSD available at the time.

In the morning Schneidermann gave a tab of LSD to everybody, and
at 7:30 p.m. police appeared at the door with a search warrant. Schneidermann's drug case, which was lying in the middle of the floor, was not ex-
amined, though Robert Fraser was caught in possession of heroin and
Jagger with four speed pills. Having just taken a bath, Faithfull
was wearing only a fur rug when police arrived, a factual tid-
bit that lead to some juicy, though never confirmed speculations (group sex, Mars bar as a sex toy, etc.). Following
a three-day trial, Richards was sentenced to a year in
prison, Jagger three months, and Fraser six months.
An outcry from the *Times* and others eventually
led to Jagger's and Richards's release on probation, and the band continued on their
way. Faithfull, who in the meantime
had been dropped, suffered for years
as a street junkie before finally making a
comeback with a newly world-weary voice.
While Keith Richards would continue to be
arrested and tried on drug charges, the more cautious
(and cleaner-living) Mick Jagger managed to avoid further
conflict despite occasional cocaine use—he had 3 grams delivered for
his wedding with Bianca Rose Perez-Mora.

THE MOST
HORRIFIC PCP STORIES

Under the influence of PCP, Carlos I. scratched his own **EYES OUT OF THEIR SOCKETS** and held them out to a police officer.

Seventeen-year-old Barry E. **BEAT** an old woman **TO DEATH**, laid down next to the body, and was unable to remember anything the next morning.

In an attempt to create a "peace pill," a Los Angeles biochemist discovered PHP, a compound similar to PCP. He swallowed the drug, undressed, climbed onto a pole, and **WAS KILLED** when a police officer, who felt threatened by the man's odd behavior, shot him six times.

A doctor gave his mother cocaine laced with PCP to treat her depression. While cleaning her house, the woman remembered that she had wanted to deposit a check at the bank across the street. She was still holding her broom when she entered the bank building. When the cashier asked about the broom, the woman held it up and told him she was **ROBBING THE BANK**.

Donald I. watched the film *J.D.'s Revenge* while high on PCP. The lead character in the film, named Ike, walks into a nightclub, where he is hypnotized. In a hypnotic trance, Ike is convinced that he is a thug named J.D. who was murdered in a slaughterhouse. Donald I. had also worked for a butcher—his father—and he identified with J.D. He had his hair cut the way the character J.D.'s was cut in the film, and when he looked in the mirror he saw J.D.'s face staring back at him. He followed a woman while carrying a pistol. Believing the pistol was the last pistol in the world, he screamed at her, **"I AM THE DEVIL!"** After shooting the passengers in a car driving by, he exchanged fire with police officers and was eventually taken into custody.

Lenny B. imagined he was flying around a duck farm. At home, he walked like a duck, quacked, and insisted he was Donald Duck. Then he **STABBED** a man to death. He was apprehended as he was splashing around in a puddle by the side of the road.

Luther P. cut off his **PENIS** and swallowed it. After medics managed to stop the bleeding, he threw up the penis. He felt no pain.

After coming home from church one Sunday, Sergio D. and his wife decided to smoke a little PCP. They turned on the TV and watched a cooking show in which the host explained how to gut and clean a fish. Sergio dozed off. He woke up to what sounded like a washing machine. When he turned to his wife, the creature standing in front of him looked like dried fish and had a black hole where the face was supposed to be. Steam was coming from the body. The voice of God told

Sergio that the creature was Satan. He cleaned Satan as if the body were a fish. Sergio, as it turned out, had **KILLED AND MUTILATED** his wife.

Martin L., seventeen, smashed windowpanes with karate kicks. When the police arrived, he attacked them with a **BUTCHER'S KNIFE**. Even after beating him several times with their batons, the police were unable to overpower Martin, who showed no signs of exhaustion or pain. In the end, it took six officers to get the better of him. The first words he spoke at the hospital were the sing-song, *"I'm strong to the finish, because I eat my spinach, I'm Popeye the sailorman."*

Some users high on PCP are said to have even managed to break out of handcuffs. Others have **CUT OFF THEIR LEGS** with an ax and then either bled to death or drowned themselves in puddles.

A FEW SONGS ON THE JOYS OF

Ecstasy

ALASTIS "Ecstasy"
BABYSHAMBLES "Hooligans on E"
BONE THUGS-N-HARMONY "Ecstasy"
BOONDOX "Rollin' Hard"
EMINEM "The Kids"
E-ROTIC "Ecstasy"
E-ZEE POSSEE "Everything Starts with an E"
FATBOY SLIM "Acid 8000"
GREEN VELVET "La La Land"
HAPPY MONDAYS "24 Hour Party People"
MAC DRE "Thizzelle Dance"
THE MAGNETIC FIELDS "Take Ecstasy with Me"
MISSY ELLIOT "4 My People"
MOBY "Next Is the E"
PAUL OAKENFOLD "Starry-Eyed Surprise"
PRIMAL SCREAM "Higher Than the Sun"
PULP "Sorted for E's and Wizz"
ROB GEE "Ecstasy, You Got What I Need"
THE SHAMEN "Ebeneezer Goode"
WARRIOR SOUL "Trippin' on Ecstasy"

FRIEND NUMBER 13

Courtney Love

Her mother accused her father of having given her LSD when she was only four years old. Though this has never been proven, it would seem an adequate prologue for a life filled with drug-infused tragedy. After a tumultuous youth and some experience as a stripper, Courtney Love (born 1964) started a few bands and dated musicians until finally meeting Nirvana singer Kurt Cobain in 1991 at the Satyricon club in Portland. They married soon after, and daughter Frances Bean Cobain was born on August 1992. A *Vanity Fair* article claimed that Love knowingly continued to use heroin even after she was pregnant, an allegation that the singer denies.

The Love-Cobain family lived in a house in the woods and chucked their own firewood—only heroin was disturbing the peace. When Cobain shot himself in 1994, Love continued to use cocaine. For years she stumbled between her critically acclaimed album releases and winning a Golden Globe for her role in *The People vs. Larry Flint* on one hand, and drug-related woes on the other. Love also claims to have been swindled out of $69 million while she "went cuckoo."

Love was arrested in 2003 for breaking the windows of her boyfriend's home and charged with possession of controlled substances. She then slapped Kurt Cobain's mother at the ensuing custody trial. Later that year she checked into rehab in California. In February 2004 *People* magazine speculated that she had "one week to live," echoing the famous *Sun* headline about Boy George. After a probation violation, Love was sentenced to twenty-eight days of lockdown rehab in August 2005.

Today she is an active Buddhist, chanting up to four hours each day. When old friends stop by for some blow, she tells them to go to hell. Whether or not she is the granddaughter of Marlon Brando (her mother's mother allegedly had an affair with him) has not been verified to date.

POPULAR 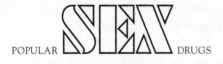 DRUGS

AMYL NITRITE (POPPERS)

★ Amyl nitrite was originally prescribed as a treatment for angina and acts as a strong vasodilator, expanding the blood vessels. It relaxes the user's muscles and produces a brief euphoric rush. Both of these characteristics make amyl nitrite a favorite for anal sex. Poppers are sold in sex shops in small, dark bottles. The name *poppers* refers to the popping noise that occurs when the bottle is opened; liquid escaping from the cap is then inhaled directly from the capsule, producing a feeling of dizziness and arousal in a matter of seconds. Effects can be felt in one to ten minutes, depending on the dose. Poppers can become especially dangerous when taken in combination with Viagra, and could result in brain damage and death. Other names: Amy, Ames, Animal, DVD Cleaner, Liquid Gold, Locker Room, Pearl, Rush, Stephen Armstrong, Snapper, TNT.

★

GHB (LIQUID ECSTASY)

★ 4-hydroxybutanoic acid, formerly gamma-hydroxybutyrate (hence the acronym), is closely related to the human neurotransmitter GABA. First synthesized in 1960, it is sometimes prescribed to prevent sleep attacks in narcoleptics. It first began to circulate as a party drug in the early 1990s. Higher doses of GHB can cause the user to slip into a coma, one reason for its common designation as the "date rape drug." In smaller doses the drug reduces inhibitions and induces a feeling of euphoria. Other names: Cherry Meth, Eclipse, Liquid X, Scoop, Serenity, Fantasy. Caution: GHB is highly corrosive.

METH, CRYSTAL METH

★ Methamphetamine increases sexual appetite and performance. Ejaculation and orgasm are either postponed or totally impossible. Raised adrenaline and dopamine levels often lead to unprotected sex, and long, vigorous sexual activity increases the risk of injuring mucous membranes. Crystal meth consumption has also contributed to the recent surge in HIV infections. Special therapies are available to former crystal meth users who, after quitting the substance, have lost all interest in sex.

VIAGRA ★

★ Was introduced to the market by the Pfizer company in 1998, putting a spark back into *Playboy* founder Hugh Hefner's sex life, among others. The active ingredient is known as Sildenafil, a substance that increases penile erection ability when aroused. Also the clitoris will become enlarged. Strangely, when taken in higher doses, sex gets a little boring. Maybe because it takes so long. Viagra should never be taken with greasy foods or combined with ecstasy—a Berlin photographer who had taken this mix once fainted in his stairwell.

TESTOSTERONE
☆ The masculine sex hormone increases sexual desire in both men and women. Testosterone no longer needs to be administered with an injection; it can also be applied as a gel or adhesive bandage or released from an implant.

TRIBULUS TERRESTRIS
☆ *Tribulus terrestris*, or Puncture Vine, is widespread in tropical and subtropical countries and is known to dramatically increase the number of sex hormone receptors. It is also popular as a natural anabolic steroid among bodybuilders.

PT-141/BREMELANOTIDE (STILL UNDER DEVELOPMENT)
☆ Doctors at an Arizona cancer center were looking for a self-tanner. During the clinical tests for Melatonin II, several of the male volunteer test subjects—including impotent ones—began experiencing spontaneous erections. Melatonin II, the active agent from which Bremelanotide was developed, increases sexual desire in men and women. The substance will be made available as a nasal spray. Side effects: flushed complexion, nausea.

VML 670
☆ Initially developed to treat nausea and as an antidepressant medication, though laboratory animals mostly showed a drastic increase in their willingness to copulate.

BUPROPION HYDROCHLORIDE
☆ Marketed in the United States as either the antidepressant Wellbutrin or Zyban, the antismoking pill. The drug decreases the need for nicotine. Users may be disgusted by cigarettes but will experience an increase in sexual appetite.

ARSENIC
☆ Was popular among Tyrolese horse handlers as early as the sixteenth century. At that time, horses were given arsenic to improve their overall condition. Europeans in the mid-eighteenth century also regularly used it for better skin, glossier hair, and (last but not least) to boost sexual energy and endurance.

YOHIMBINE
☆ A white powder derived from the dried bark extract of the West African yohimbe tree. Causes a dramatic dilation of the blood vessels and promotes blood circulation—also to the loins. Can have a psychedelic effect in higher doses; the body seems to be "melting." Undesirable side effects: excessive sweating, dizziness, nausea, heart palpitations, and low blood pressure.

DAMIANA
☆ Damiana (*Turnera diffusa*) is a flowering shrub native to Central America and Mexico; early users include the Mayans, who took it as both an aphrodisiac and a pick-me-up. The leaves of the plant have a stimulating, antidepressive effect (they also contain caffeine) and have been known to increase skin sensitivity. In Mexico, Damiana is scientifically recognized as a treatment for sexual impotence and spermatorrhea (involuntary ejaculation).

CATUABA

☆ A pharmacological analysis of the Brazilian tree bark detected phytosterols, a chemical component similar to sexual hormones and attributed cause of catuaba's potency-enhancing effects. Experienced users of the substance swear by it.

ELEUTHEROCOCCUS SENTICOSUS
☆ Not a sex drug in the strictest sense but an overall fitness booster that can help when taken in combination with other substances. Studies conducted with bodybuilders, wrestlers, and gymnasts showed an increase in performance ability, decreased exhaustion, and improved mood. Healthy athletes showed increased endurance, along with lowered lactate levels (a parameter for body oxygen metabolism) and sustained lower blood pressure (a stress parameter).

APOMORPHINE
☆ Apomorphine was once used as a vomit inducer in cases of poisoning. As Uprima it is a best-selling erectile dysfunction drug in Europe and is under investigation in the United States and Canada. The medication promotes dopamine production, and some sources claim that it is also effective for women. Its effects appear to be something of a double-edged sword, however; 10% stop taking it due to nausea and vomiting.

CANNABIS
☆ Aside from the occasional cannabis-induced paranoia attack, the biggest danger with this aphrodisiac is becom-

Sex Cocktail,
EASY TO MAKE AND COMPLETELY LEGAL

THE INGREDIENTS
★ 250 grams catuaba root, 1 liter ethanol. The alcohol draws phytosterols from the root. Allow to sit for fourteen days in a dark broom closet. If no ethanol is available (or too expensive), then schnapps will do the trick. When the mixture is ready, pour it through a coffee filter. Now the phytosterols are in your glass; 0.1 cl per use is enough.
★ 30 to 60 Damiana drops. Ask at your local homeopathic pharmacy or health food store.
★ 30 to 60 drops Yohombine. Available in liquid form as a dietary supplement—check health food stores.
★ 0.01 cl Eleuterococcus. Also known as Siberian Ginseng, available in health food stores and homeopathic pharmacies.
DIRECTIONS FOR USE
Drink in one gulp and in thirty to sixty minutes you're ready to go.
A mighty erection will appear and skin will become very sensitive.

ing overly relaxed and simply falling asleep. To prevent this, users in the Arabic world often combine their hashish with coffee. Talking to *Newsweek* in the 1960s, renowned psychiatrist Dr. Nathan Kline warned that users under the influence of marijuana "love everyone" and may be more inclined to promiscuity, making pregnancy "one of the most common side effects of pot." Cannabis lowers testosterone levels—in the seventies, budget-minded transsexuals used it as a low-cost hormone therapy, though to no avail.

FIGGING

☆ Ginger or chili is either inserted into the anus or vagina or rubbed into the penis, guaranteeing a sustained burning sensation and improved blood circulation. In the old days, ginger was inserted into a horse's anus when he went to market, so that the horse would appear livelier and hold its tail high. The English expression "to gin up" is purportedly derived from this practice.

WORLDWIDE

ECSTASY SEIZURES

Australia	27% 1,436
USA	14% 748
Netherlands	12% 627
United Kingdom	9% 499
Canada	6% 321
Belgium	5% 255
China	4% 234
Turkey	3% 175
Germany	3% 159
Malaysia	2% 106
Ireland	2% 88
Hungary	2% 85
France	2% 83
Spain	57
Japan	52
Poland	49
Italy	40
Dominican Republic	28
Taiwan, Prov. of China	27
Israel	27

Seizures of ecstasy in kilogram equivalents and in % of world total.

Data from 2005. *Source:* UN 2007 World Drug Report

GLAMOROUS

REHAB CLINICS

◎ HAZELDEN—Founded in 1949, the main center is idyllically located on a Minnesota lakeside. Author James Frey griped about his experiences there in his not-completely-authentic memoir, *A Million Little Pieces*. Other former guests include Liza Minelli, Calvin Klein, and Melanie Griffith. The center's homepage features esoteric food for thought and sells a glass pendant engraved with a camel and the words *"Expect miracles of change in people's lives."*

◎ PROMISES—The Malibu branch offers "a gorgeous panoramic view of the Pacific Ocean." Patients have included Diana Ross, Winona Ryder, and Ben Affleck. Interested guests may also opt for a therapy that includes horses; the English *Independent* called it "psychobabble in a saddle." Robert Downey Jr.'s publicist said to *W* in 2002: *"Obviously it didn't work for him."*

◎ PRIORY CLINIC—The England-based Priory group claims to be "Europe's leading independent provider of acute mental health, secure and step-down services . . . , [and] neuro-rehabilitation services." Founded in 1872, the clinic is London's oldest psychiatric hospital. Treatment methods include EMDR (eye

movement desensitization and reprocessing). English soccer player Paul Gascoigne, singer Sinéad O'Connor, Johnny Depp, and Ron Wood of the Rolling Stones stayed there for a time.

◎ PASSAGES—Founded by bestselling author Chris Prentiss (*The Little Book of Secrets: 81 Secrets for Enjoying a Happy, Prosperous, and Successful Life*) and his formerly heroin-addicted son Pax. The Malibu clinic claims to have the lowest relapse rate of all, which experts are inclined to dispute. Residents enjoy a Koi carp pond, a twelve-foot-tall Statue of Liberty replica on the lawn and a chef who developed two dressings for the actor Paul Newman's Newman's Own series.

◎ THAMKRABOK—Thai Buddhist monastery located 100 miles north of Bangkok. The hundred monks and twenty nuns who live there have been helping recovering opium addicts since 1961. Director Luang Phoo Tscharoen has created music based on shapes found in nature and practices a special glass-painting technique. The therapy itself is considered particularly harsh: The addict has to drink a plant extract that causes violent vomiting for the first five days, and constant meditation is highly recommended. British musician Pete Doherty (Babyshambles) tried to kick his heroin addiction here. Treatment is free, but donations are gladly accepted.

◎ BEAU MONDE—*"The greater the star power, the more complex the problems"* says clinic director Heidi Kunzli. For every guest there are fifteen employees, including traditional healers and personal fitness trainers; amenities include lava rock massage. A minimum stay at this Malibu clinic is two weeks.

◎ BETTY FORD CENTER—Founded by the former First Lady in 1982 following her own battles with breast cancer and alcohol and pill addiction. The thirty-day standard therapy costs $21,000. There are a number of branches. The main campus is located in Rancho Mirage, California, and is rather modestly decorated. Numerous celebrity patients have included Liza Minelli, Ali MacGraw, William Hurt, Don Johnson, Billy Joel, Drew Barrymore, Johnny Cash, and Keith Urban. This is also where Liz Taylor met her seventh husband, construction worker Larry Fortensky. How he was able to afford the therapy remains unclear.

◎ THE MEADOWS/ARIZONA— Picturesque location in Arizona's beautiful Sonoran Desert, with a primary focus on the common addictions: alcohol, drugs, and medication. And sex: Meadows consultant Pia Mellody authored the books *Facing Love Addiction* and *The Intimacy Factor*. The Meadows treats, "compulsive use of cybersex, use of prosti-

tutes, and exposing oneself," among other problems. Kate Moss checked in here to treat her cocaine addiction. T-shirts with suggestive slogans are prohibited—all major credit cards accepted.

◎ SILVER HILL HOSPITAL—The New Canaan, Connecticut, hospital has been treating neuroses and addictions since 1931. Patients have included Liza Minelli, Truman Capote, and Nick Nolte. They live in Tudor cottages, and the house rules are rigid: no laptops, and packages must be opened under supervision. Mariah Carey checked in here when she heard the voice of Marilyn Monroe coming out of her piano.

◎ SIERRA TUCSON—The medical stabilization program costs $2,100 per day at first; later on it gets cheaper. Therapeutic methods range from classic to novel, and include psychodrama, EMDR, somatic trauma therapy, qi gong, and Native American talking circles. Low-fat desserts are served twice a week. Clients have included Rob Lowe, Ringo Starr, and Michael Douglas.

◎ CROSSROADS CENTRE—This rehab clinic is nestled on the Caribbean island of Antigua, known for its captivating landscape. It was founded by Eric Clapton in 1998—notice that his 1998 CD box set also bears the same name. A former junkie and alcoholic himself, Clapton ("If you wanna get down, down to the ground: cocaine") is a particularly believable sobriety advocate. The standard treatment runs at about $21,500, plus a $500 deposit for medical expenses.

PSYCHEDELIC CHURCHES

The following churches were founded in the United States and Canada starting at the end of the nineteenth century. Each of them either once involved or currently involves partaking of psychoactive sacraments:

Native American Church—Peyote

Church of the First Born—Peyote

Church of the Awakening—Peyote

Ghost Clan—Peyote

Peyote Way Church—Peyote

League for Spiritual Discovery—LSD

Original Kleptonian Neo-American Church—LSD, Peyote

Paleo-American Church—Assorted varieties

Church of the Golden Rule—Assorted varieties

Church of the Sunshine—Assorted varieties

Psychedelic Peace Fellowship—Assorted varieties

Universal Life Church—Assorted varieties

Dog Commune—LSD

Shivalia—LSD

Church of the Tree of Light—DMT

Church of the One Sermon—Psilo mushrooms

Fane of the Psilocybe Mushroom Association—Psilo mushrooms

Temple of the True Inner Light—DPT

Religion of Drugs—LSD

New American Church—LSD

Church of the Psychedelic Mystic—Assorted varieties

Church of the Toad of Light—Bufo avarius (Colorado river toad) glandular secretions

Church of the North American Shaman—Assorted varieties

Inter-Faith Assembly of the Psychedelic Church of God—Assorted varieties

First International Church of Salvia Divinorum—Salvia divinorum

International Copelandia Church of God—Copelandia mushrooms

Church of Gnostic Luminism—Assorted varieties

Shiva Fellowship Church—LSD, Cannabis

Psychedelic Venus Church—Cannabis

Church of All Worlds—Opium, Cannabis

Our Church—Cannabis

First Hawaiian Church of the Holy Smoke—Cannabis

Religion of Jesus Church—Cannabis

Children of the Mist Church—Cannabis

Church of Cognizance—Cannabis

HOW TO RECOGNIZE WHICH DRUGS
A PERSON HAS TAKEN BASED ON THEIR
APPEARANCE

The following well-known symptoms appear to varying degrees and are dependent upon dosage and other circumstances. Diagnosis becomes considerably more complicated in cases where different drugs have been mixed.

<u>WITHOUT DRUGS</u>
(for comparison)

<u>COCAINE</u>
- Teeth grinding
- Constant, repeated sniffing
- Fidgeting with nose
- Nose bleeds
- White crumbs around nostrils, sometimes also a small white patch
- Frequent trips to the toilet
- Long fingernails (as a sign of their rejection of physical labor—these are also useful for arranging the cocaine on a mirror or scooping the powder into the nose)
- Skin picked away from the fingernails
- Increase sweating, even while sitting or lying down
- Dry, scaly skin

<u>SPEED</u>
- Teeth grinding
- Constant, repeated sniffing
- Fidgeting with nose
- Nose bleeds
- White crumbs around nostrils, sometimes also a small white patch
- Frequent trips to the toilet
- Skin picked away from the fingernails
- Increased sweating, even while sitting or lying down
- Dry, scaly skin
- Trembling
- Senseless routines

<u>ALCOHOL</u>
- Boozy breath/alcoholic fetor (approximately 20% of consumed alcohol is exhaled by the lungs)
- Babbling
- Impaired motor skills
- Aggression
- Sentimentality
- Lowered inhibitions
- Red face
- After years of drinking: "drinker's nose"/ rhinophyma (bulbous-like growth of the nose is presumably caused by growth hormones in the liver that cannot be processed quickly enough)

HEROIN
- White, doughy skin
- Slowed speech and movements, as if paralyzed
- Pin-sized pupils
- Injection scars or "track marks" on the forearm or in other areas of the body where veins are visible
- Malnourishment (sunken eyes, protruding cheekbones)

ECSTASY
- Dilated pupils
- Jaw clenching
- Restlessness
- Constant grin
- Sensual movements
- Need for physical closeness
- Reddened, sometimes blotchy face

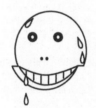

CANNABIS
- Bloodshot eyes (due to a drop in intraocular pressure)
- Eyes half closed
- Grinning
- Senseless laughter
- Lethargy
- Paleness (blood circulation to the skin and outer extremities is slowed)
- Squinting (THC hinders the ability to produce tears)

POPULAR

OPIUM PRESCRIPTIONS IN WORLD HISTORY

EBERS PAPYRUS (SIXTEENTH CENTURY B.C.)
⊙ The Egyptian Ebers papyrus, one of the world's oldest medical documents, contains a remedy for quieting screaming children. The prescription calls for wasp dung and "mehes" seed capsules, which probably refers to poppy.

THERIAC (SECOND CENTURY B.C.)
⊙ Theriac is a mixture containing up to three hundred various, often interchangeable ingredients such as duck's blood, bear bile, crawfish, kummel, and rennet, but most importantly opium, garden angelica (*Angelica sylvestris*), real valeriana, and carrot seed (*Daucus carota*). Theriac was an antidote originally developed by Greek doctors, and at first it contained only ingredients such as viper flesh, various herbs and roots, honey, and wine. The first to add opium was Andromache, personal physician to the Roman emperor Nero. Theriac was extremely popular in antiquity. Consumption slowed in old Rome after the spread of Christianity but blossomed soon after in the Arabic world. At banquets, the

Caliph Al-Mutawakkil would entertain dinner guests by allowing himself to be bitten by poisonous snakes and treating the bite with theriac afterward. Theriac was used up to the sixteenth century as an all-purpose miracle cure against pests, syphilis, and witchcraft. The medical school in Paris recommended theriac with every meal. Its preparation was made into a festival in some parts of Italy.

MITHRIDATE, MITHRIDATIUM (CA. 100 B.C.)

⊙ Mithrides VI Eupator, King of Pontus, had a constant fear of being poisoned. As a precaution he took a daily slug of his own toxic brew containing various poisons, among them venom, arsenic, alraune, henbane, and opium. The altogether forty- to fifty-ingredient concoction was actually called *athanasia*. Mithridates VI became the victim of his own preventative measure after he was conquered by the Roman military leader Pompey. His self-poisoning attempt failed and he was forced to make a soldier stab him to death instead. Pompey found Mithridates's recipe and had it translated into Latin. "Mithridatium" became an important part of Roman society.

SLEEP SPONGE (NINTH CENTURY)

⊙ A sponge is soaked in numbing, calming plant extracts (opium, cow parsley, alraune) and held up to the nostrils. This was used as a general anesthesia in the Middle Ages; sleep sponges were even used in fourteenth-century brain tumor surgeries.

SMUDGING (SIXTEENTH CENTURY)

⊙ Heinrich Agrippa von Nettesheim (1486–1535), probably the inspiration behind the character Doctor Faustus, recommended using incense, or smudging, as a way of making ghosts perceivable—with black poppy, alraune, henbane, and cat's brain.

LAUDANUM (SIXTEENTH CENTURY)

⊙ Theophrastus Bombastus von Hohenheim (1493–1541), also known as Paracelsus, invented this concoction consisting of 90% alcohol (wine) and 10% opium and henbane. In Europe, laudanum was a very popular pain reliever and tranquilizer until the nineteenth century, when it also gained popularity as a hallucinogen. The substance is still available by prescription in the United States, classified as a Schedule II drug under the Controlled Substances Act.

L'EAU HÉROIQUE (SEVENTEENTH CENTURY)

⊙ Composed of coffee, opium, and camphor. Prince Eugene of Savoy (1663–1736), a French commander who fought for Austria, brought it back from the Turkish Wars.

DOVER'S POWDER (EIGHTEENTH CENTURY)

⊙ Powder developed by English doctor Thomas Dover. The preparation consisting of opium, potassium carbonate, and ipecacuanha was used against oncoming fever.

PAREGORIC (EIGHTEENTH CENTURY)

⬤ Composed of alcohol, opium (later morphine), camphor, and anise oil. Paregoric slows the digestive tract and was used in the United States to control fulminant diarrhea. John F. Kennedy took it regularly.

BLACK DROP (NINETEENTH CENTURY)

⬤ Composed of opium, vinegar, yeast, and spices that included psychoactive nutmeg. The English poet Samuel Taylor Coleridge ("Xanadu") used Black Drop to treat his rheumatoid arthritis: "*In an evil hour I procured it: it worked miracles—the swellings disappeared, the pains vanished. I was all alive, and all around me being as ignorant as myself, nothing could exceed my triumph. I talked of nothing else, prescribed the newly discovered panacea for all complaints, and carried a little about with me not to lose any opportunity of administering 'instant relief and speedy cure' to all complainers, stranger or friend, gentle or simple. Alas! it is with a bitter smile, a laugh of gall and bitterness, that I recall this period of unsuspecting delusion, and how I first became aware of the Maelstrom, the fatal whirlpool to which I was drawing.*"

MOTHER BAILEY'S QUIETING SYRUP (NINETEENTH CENTURY)

⬤ In the early days of industrialization, low wages forced women working in Manchester textile mills to leave their unattended children at home. To calm them, children were given the opium-containing Mother Bailey's or similar products such as Dr. McMunn's Elixir, Godfrey's Cordial, Street's Infants' Quietness, Atkinson's, Infants' Preservative, Squire's Elixir, Mrs. Winslow's Soothing Syrup, Daffy's Elixir, Battley's Sedative Solution, Batley's Drops, Kendal Black Drops, or Dalby's Carminative.

HOW TO RECOGNIZE

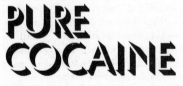
PURE COCAINE

✖ Rub a small amount between your fingers and the crystals will dissolve at body temperature. Good cocaine will feel oily.

✖ A bit of cocaine can be heated with a lighter on a sheet of aluminum foil.

It should melt and evaporate but not burn, leaving only a little spot with a lacquer-like consistency. Wipe it with your finger and your finger should come up clean.

✖ Color is unimportant, as it depends entirely on the drying technique. White cocaine is dried in the sun, yellow under strong lamps.

✖ Poured in a glass of lukewarm water, finely chopped cocaine should dissolve in the upper third of the glass. Nothing should settle at the bottom.

FRIEND NUMBER 14
Whitney Houston

Her former sister-in-law must really hate her: Tina
Brown, sister to Houston's ex-husband Bobby, never
misses a chance to tattle on the singer's private
life. In spring 2006, Brown publicly disclosed the
singer's problems in a tell-all exclusive for the
National Enquirer: Photos showed the singer's
Atlanta bathroom littered with crack pipes,
cocaine-coated spoons, cigarette butts, Budweiser cans, and garbage, to which Brown also
delivered the sordid details of Houston's bizarre hab-
its: hallucinating demons, biting and hitting herself, punching
through walls, and locking herself away with her crack pipe and an impressive array of sex toys.

Whitney Houston's (born 1963) career began in 1985 with a fabulously successful
debut album and a squeaky-clean image. With record sales topping 170 million, the
former gospel singer recorded six chart-topping studio albums and three hit movie
soundtracks, including *The Bodyguard*, which ranks as the best-selling soundtrack of
all time. Houston's glittering persona slowly corroded after her marriage to Bobby
Brown in 1992, when rumors of drug addiction, eating disorders, and domestic violence grew louder.

In January 2000, shortly before Houston's *Greatest Hits* album release, the
couple was caught toting a half ounce of marijuana in their luggage at a Hawaii
airport. Houston did not appear in court; she instead sent two lawyers and the
negative results of a voluntarily submitted drug test. Sentence: a $2,100 dona-
tion to an antidrug program for youth and three months on probation.

The troubled singer was fired from her Oscar performance that same
year. Just months later, employees at the Grandover Resort in North Carolina found an empty bottle of Jack Daniels, sixteen empty bottles of beer,
a bag of marijuana, and a plastic bag containing baking powder in Suite
1114. The baking powder was taken as proof that Houston had been pre-
paring crack. *"Crack is whack,"* she famously responded in her 2002 interview with Diane Sawyer, *"I make too much money to smoke crack."* She did,
however, admit that she *"partied her tail off."*

Somehow her life never seemed to settle down. At the Ocean Club Resort
in 2003, Bobby Brown flirted with Spice Girl Emma Bunton and Houston angrily
confronted him back in their suite. A friend saw Brown grab Whitney from behind and start to choke her. Fearing for her life, Houston cracked him on the skull
with a heavy ashtray.

In 2004 she checked into a drug rehabilitation center, and by June her mood had improved: giggling hysterically, Houston sashayed through Harrods department store in London with her husband. Staff reported that the couple appeared "drugged and disheveled" and demanded to be given designer clothing for free.

The TV reality show *Being Bobby Brown*, which showcased the couple's home life, could be seen as the all-time low point of her career. Houston and Brown took outrageous pleasure in discussing their body functions ("I have to poop a poop") and the jittery Houston once locked their daughter out of her room so she could have sex with her husband.

Houston filed for divorce in April 2007.

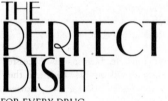

THE PERFECT DISH

FOR EVERY DRUG

❋ <u>HEROIN</u>—Regular heroin users can tolerate only very little food. Junkies tend to subsist on yogurt and strawberry milk.

❋ <u>CANNABIS</u>—Smoking a strong joint whets the appetite for sweet and greasy dishes. Chocolate bars are wolfed down whole in seconds flat. Creamier ice cream brands such as Ben & Jerry's or Häagen-Dazs are ideal, though half a leftover cheesecake from the fridge will also do in a pinch.

❋ <u>COCAINE</u>—Eating on cocaine is generally unappealing, though the morning after is a different story. What is striking is the need for hearty, down-home cooking such as pot roast, crab cakes, or steak and french fries. On the one hand, this is because many hours have passed since your last meal. On the other hand, comfort foods help compensate for feelings of loneliness caused by the drug.

❋ <u>ECSTASY</u>—The drug was initially developed as an appetite suppressant, so really all you need after taking ecstasy is lots of water. Some clubs in the nineties would remove the faucets from their sinks so that ravers would be forced to buy water at the bar—a risky move, considering dehydration can be fatal.

❋ <u>LSD</u>—Dextrose, minerals, and vitamins, especially in the form of fruit juices. Because LSD increases brain activity over the course of several hours, it stands to reason that nutritional recommendations are similar to that of a marathon runner. In the late 1960s, Dutchman Bart Hughes recommended one pound of sugar per trip.

❋ <u>SPEED</u>—Because appetite suppressants frequently contain amphetamines (speed), the question is moot. Permanent speed consumption is an effective, though not particularly healthy, weight-loss diet.

John F. Kennedy's

DRUG COCKTAIL

His rectum was *"plenty red,"* he wrote to his friend Le Moyne Billings after having been treated in the New Haven Hospital in the winter of 1934. *"Yours would be red too if you had shoved every thing from rubber tubes to iron pipe up it."* Doctors feared he might have leukemia due to his weight loss and nasty case of hives. Since childhood, John F. Kennedy had suffered from a weak constitution and digestional problems. It seems that he was treated with corticosteroids since 1937, which would have compounded his later constant back pain and the Addison's disease. As Robert Dallek points out in his book *An Unfinished Life: John F. Kennedy, 1917–1963*, the politician always wore a corset brace and had to take long hot baths to ease the pain before going to bed.

In 1955, Kennedy consulted Janet Ravell, who kept a record of his medications. At the White House, the president was under the care of an allergist, an endrocrinologist, a gastroenterologist, an orthopedist, a urologist, and Max Jacobson, aka "Dr. Feelgood," who was known for treating celebrities with amphetamines. In the first six months of his presidency he suffered from stomach, colon, and prostate problems; high fevers; abcesses; sleeplessness; high cholesterol; and back and adrenal ailments. He was prescribed corticosteroids for adrenal insufficiency; procaine shots for his back; Lomotil, Metamucil, and Paregoric (morphine, camphor, and anise oil); Phenobarbital (a barbiturate), testosterone, and trasentine for his diarrhea; penicillin for his urinary tract infections; and Tuinal (a mix of barbiturates) for his sleeplessness.

After the Cuban Missile Crisis in November 1962, Jackie Kennedy asked her husband's gastroenterologist to give him something against the "depressing action" the antihistamines had on the president. For two days he took the antipsychotic medication Stelazine.

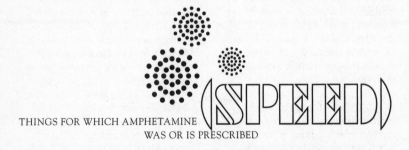

THINGS FOR WHICH AMPHETAMINE (SPEED)
WAS OR IS PRESCRIBED

🏵 Alcoholism 🏵 Anxiety 🏵 Asthma 🏵 Circulatory collapse
🏵 Encephalitis lethargica (aka sleeping sickness) 🏵 Hyperkinetic syndrome
🏵 Neuroses 🏵 Obesity 🏵 Pain 🏵 Parkinson's disease 🏵 Tiredness

SMUGGLING TRICKS

Caution: Smuggling drugs is illegal, and offenders are heavily prosecuted. None of these tricks is a safe bet.

TRAIN
◆ Wrap the drugs in aluminum foil and tuck the pack into the little trash bin in your section or take it into the bathroom, deposit it in the trash there, and retrieve it just before arrival at your destination. The biggest danger in both cases is the trash collector.

THE SURGEONS
◆ Drug dealers apparently specialize in extreme transport methods. Couriers' thigh muscles are cut open, a cocaine bag is deposited inside, and the wound is stitched up again. Disadvantage: Transported amounts tend to be rather small.

BEHIND THE BALLS
◆ Secured with strong adhesive bandage, a few grams of heroin or cocaine can be transported between the sphincter and scrotum. For private use only, due to the smallness of the stash.

MAIL WITH NO SENDER
◆ Mail a letter or package containing opium (Asia) or cocaine (South America) with no return address to a neutral location—for example, a cooperating entrepreneur's business address. Has a tendency to go awry.

BOBBEL/COLOMBIAN WEENIE
◆ Involves swallowing a cocaine- or heroin-filled condom. Couriers are called "body packers." The movie *Maria Full of Grace* depicts this practice: The protagonist carries sixty-two packets in her stomach next to her unborn child. The pain is as excruciating as the risk is high: If a portion leaks, the carrier dies of an overdose.

FABERGÉ EGG
◆ Kate Moss, according to tabloid daily the *Sun*, has repeatedly smuggled drugs in a Fabergé egg. These eggs were originally produced by jeweler Carl Peter Fabergé for the Russian czarina Maria Fyodorovna.

INDIAN RELIGIOUS OBJECTS
◆ Because of the high value placed on religious freedom in the United States, Indians flying from the southern part of the country use ritual objects, which are hollow on the inside, to smuggle drugs. Customs does not check these for fear of being sued.

CREATIVE IDEAS
◆ The imagination, of course, is limitless. There have also been reports of clothing soaked in liquid cocaine and cocaine that has been pressed into a coffee bean shape and spray-painted brown ("Colombian coffee").

OPIUM SMUGGLING:

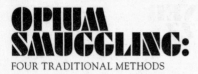

FOUR TRADITIONAL METHODS

Zhan Saiming, a clerk at an opium factory in ancient Hong Kong, listed the following methods:

☝ ON THE BODY

The typical Chinese man will smuggle opium in his cap, has a pouch filled with the substance secured under each arm and around the backsides of his thighs, has packets reinforcing his calves, and wears an opium-filled belt around his belly and a little net with opium packets between his legs.

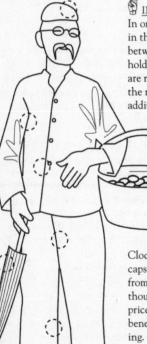

✌ IN LUGGAGE

In one hand he holds an umbrella concealing opium, in the other a basket with the tea kettle; opium lies between the basket lining and the weave. Otherwise he holds a basket full of eggs where only the eggs on top are real, the others filled with opium. False bottoms in the remaining boxes and cases he is carrying conceal an additional abundance of the substance.

🤟 WOMEN

Women are the most notorious smugglers because they are never checked. Fake breasts and a large, opium-filled pouch simulating pregnancy are especially popular with this group.

🖐 OTHER

Clockwork is removed from a pocket watch and the capsule filled with opium, or pits and meat are removed from lychee fruits and opium is packed inside. Even though the fruit is no larger than a cherry, high opium prices make it worth the trouble. On ships it's concealed beneath the planks of the deck and behind cabin paneling. Otherwise it's thrown overboard in a preferably inconspicuous casing, to be fished out again later.

STONER JAZZ

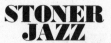

FROM THE EARLY TWENTIETH CENTURY

Kansas Joe and Memphis Minnie: "I'm Wild about My Stuff"
McKinney Cotton Pickers: "Selling That Stuff"
Cleo Brown: "The Stuff Is Here and It's Mellow"
Lil Johnson: "Mellow Stuff"
Cedar Creek Sheik: "Don't Credit My Stuff"
Oscar's Chicago Swingers: "Try Some of That"
Buck Washington: "Save the Roach for Me"
Baron Lee & the Blue Rhythm Band: "The Reefer Man"
Larry Adler: "Smoking Reefers"
Jazz Gillum & His Jazz Boys: "Reefer Head Woman"
Slim & Slam: "Dopey Joe"
Cab Calloway: "The Ghost of Smokey Joe"
Richard Jones & His Jazz Wizards: "Blue Reefer Blues"
Frankie Jaxon: "Jive Man Blues"
Don Rodman & Orchestra: "Chant of the Weed"
The Harlem Hamfats: "Weed Smokers Dream"
Bea Foote: "Weed"
The Melton Boys: "Mary Jane"
Original New Orleans Rhythm Kings: "Golden Leaf Strut"
Julia Lee & Her Boyfriends: "Spinach Song"
Stuff Smith & His Onyx Club Boys: "You're a Viper"
Mezz Mezzrow & His Orchestra: "Sendin' the Vipers"
Fats Waller: "Vipers Drag"
Sidney Bechet with Noble Sissle's Swingers: "Viper Mad"
Bob Howard & His Boys: "If You're a Viper"
The Ink Spots: "That Cat Is High"
Chick Webb & His Orchestra: "When I Get Low I Get High"
Gene Krupa and His Orchestra: "Feelin' High and Happy"
Louis Armstrong: "Kickin' the Gong Around"
Jean Brady & Big Bill Broonzy: "Knockin' Myself Out"
Trixie Smith: "Jack I'm Mellow"
Champion Jack Dupree: "Junker's Blues"
Bukka White: "Fixin' to Die Blues"
Herbert Payne: "Smoke Clouds"
Benny Goodman & His Orchestra: "Texas Tea Party"
Louis Armstrong: "Muggles"

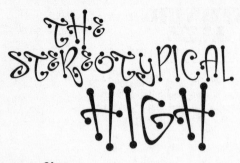

THE STEREOTYPICAL HIGH

COCAINE

- ✳ *"I'm not just saying this because I'm on coke."*
- ✳ Burning desire to tell the truth. Popular topics: old conflicts, loneliness, general coldness.
- ✳ Strong conviction that conversation is the answer.
- ✳ Talking in the bathroom and can't leave.
- ✳ Strong urge to have sex but can't get an erection.
- ✳ Keep drinking alcohol but never get drunk.
- ✳ Saliva tastes bitter, gums go numb.
- ✳ Belief that everything is under control while taking more and more, faster and faster.
- ✳ Insomnia: *"Should I take some more or am I falling asleep now? But that's not how it works."*
- ✳ Depression afterward.

HEROIN

- ✳ Few to no words.
- ✳ Feeling of warmth and languidness, coupled with a cold superiority toward the rest of the world.
- ✳ Other people coolly, clearly observed,

almost inspected.
- ✳ Sex is possible, though not especially interesting. Heroin users are enough in themselves.
- ✳ The user is surrounded by an aura of untouchability.

ECSTASY

- ✳ *"I really feel it now."*
- ✳ *"Man, I'm out of it."*
- ✳ *"You've got such nice ears, can I touch them?"*
- ✳ Touching and stroking so long that sex is forgotten.
- ✳ You forget to drink.
- ✳ Warmth, softness, smiling.
- ✳ Clear, pure euphoria: every sensual perception rediscovered, truly felt for the first time and more intensely than ever before.

LSD

- ✳ *"I don't feel anything . . ."* and after a few minutes: *". . . oh, now it's starting."*
- ✳ A few hours later: *"How long 'til this wears off?"*
- ✳ *"The floor is so three-dimensional."*
- ✳ *"Do you see the same thing when you*

close your eyes?"

✳ *"Oh my God, look what's happening to the wall."*

✳ On the street, in the subway: You become acutely worried that others can tell how completely differently you are walking and looking around. You pull yourself together, deliberately and mechanically look from left to right, slowly walk pulling one foot after the other. This is a tedious process, but one that fills you with contentment and pride.

✳ No matter how fast you are moving, it is not as fast as it feels. You feel like a regular lightning bolt.

✳ The field of vision appears to be expanding. A little light, way off to the right, colors the entire visual area. The longer you look at something, the more radically it changes. Sex is therefore an extremely delicate matter; anything repetitive and monotone and suddenly you're gone—far away from the other person but also from yourself. In only a few seconds time you are suddenly a completely different being in a strange space.

✳ It's all a matter of concentration.

CANNABIS

✳ *"Uhh . . . fingers . . . !"* while slowly moving your hand in front of your face.

✳ The initial rush is replaced by a languorous, inevitable need to be calm and say nothing.

✳ You get cozy, roll your shoulders forward, and cuddle up to yourself. *"Leave us alone, we just wanna chill."*

✳ In higher doses: Unlike alcohol,

where tunnel vision is only experienced, here you feel it too. The field of vision is for the most part a grayish black, and light and shapes are only in the middle.

✳ Just focusing on something makes it feel closer. A slight focal shift makes it slip back into the distance. The room billows slightly.

✳ Having sex could mean sliding very far down. Better to keep the eyes open so as not to forget where you are and how everything fits together anatomically and personally.

✳ Constant frustration in two-person conversations because the other person is just grinning, half looking past you, only blankly glances up every now and again, and is very obviously neither listening to nor understanding what you're saying. If you listen to yourself, you notice that you lost your train of thought long ago and also have no idea what you were talking about.

KETAMINE

✳ *"My legs are about fifteen feet long and so elastic."*

✳ The body seems to be wringing itself out.

✳ *"Can I still feel my body at all?"*

✳ Field of vision looks like wavy sheet metal at the edges.

✳ Layers of time are shifted and convoluted: past, present, and future are no longer clearly separable.

✳ You're dancing as if on autopilot with no sense of space or time—in a "k hole."

✳ Afterward: *"I can't remember anything."*

FRIEND NUMBER 15
Stephen King

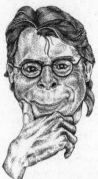

"Creative people probably do run a greater risk of alcoholism and addiction than those in some other jobs, but so what? We all look pretty much the same when we're puking in the gutter," he said. The best-selling author admitted to having based the character of Jack Torrance, an ex-alcoholic who falls under the spell of a haunted hotel in *The Shining*, on himself.

King was addicted to cocaine from 1979 to 1987, described the drug as his "on switch," and claimed that it saved him from dying of alcoholism. At some point his wife dumped his trash out in front of him to reveal *"beer cans, cigarette butts, cocaine in gram bottles and cocaine in plastic baggies, coke spoons caked with snot and blood, Valium, Xanax, bottles of Robitussin cough syrup and NyQuil cold medicine, even bottles of mouthwash."* Stephen King (born 1947) gave up most of the drugs in the late eighties but is still a loyal fan of the least harmful one: *"I think that marijuana should not only be legal, I think it should be a cottage industry. It would be wonderful for the state of Maine. There's some pretty good homegrown dope. I'm sure it would be even better if you could grow it with fertilizers and have greenhouses."* King does not remember a number of books he wrote under the influence.

THE BIGGEST
DRUG GATHERINGS

BURNING MAN
● Multitoxic New Age festival in Sierra Nevada. Nearly 40,000 annual visitors dedicate themselves to the search for meaning, shamanism, symbolic art, and self-drummed music. Very important: Dispose of your own trash. Drugs: mushrooms, mescaline, LSD, ecstasy.

GAY PRIDE
● Homosexuals the world over celebrate Christopher Street Day (June 27), the day in which New York City gays resisted police persecution and discrimination in 1967. Among the drugs keeping the party both long and wild: ecstasy, cocaine, and poppers.

FULL MOON PARTY
● Practiced anywhere with enough hippies and sun, wherever barefoot dancing is allowed. Ko Phangan, Thailand; Ibiza; Atacama Desert, Chile. Drugs: yaba, ecstasy, speed.

LOVE PARADE
● Berlin summer block party steeped in tradition, followed by countless after-parties in local clubs. The Love Parade first took place in 1989 with 150 participants, has grown steadily with every passing year, and has inspired copycat parties around the world. 1.5 million visitors visited Berlin in 1999. Constant fights with city authorities and flagging public interest caused the parade to move to Essen in 2007. Any drug goes—the classic is ecstasy.

GLASTONBURY FESTIVAL
● Open-air concert at which many a British celebrity has cultivated their drug image: Robbie Williams infamously partied with Oasis here after being kicked out of his band Take That, Primal Scream frontman Bobbie Gillespie addressed the audience as *"fucking hippies,"* and Kate Moss strutted through the muck with her Pete Doherty. Drugs: everything.

MIAMI WINTER MUSIC CONFERENCE
● The alleged industry gathering with panels, workshops, and product innovations is actually a five-day-long South Beach party, held every year in March. There's no holding out with Red Bull alone. Preferred drugs: amphetamine, ecstasy.

STONY AWARDS
● Culture prize ceremony initiated by *High Times* magazine, honoring films devoted to cannabis diffusion and glorification. Past winners include *A Scanner Darkly* and the series *Weeds* in 2006. Field research is awarded at the Cannabis Cup in Amsterdam, a trade fair at which new marijuana strains are introduced and awarded prizes.

OKTOBERFEST
● The carefully crafted image of a rustic Volksfest isn't really all that fitting. Several celebrities have been caught using cocaine to help the copious amounts of wheat beer go down easier.

ART BASEL MIAMI BEACH
● Very successful offshoot of the world's most influential contemporary art fair. Art Basel Miami enjoys the reputation of being more party- than business-oriented. Drugs: You're in Miami!

PROMINENT

VIN MARIANI DRINKERS

The French cocaine-and-wine tonic had many friends in the nineteenth century, among them:
Sarah Bernhardt
Alexandre Dumas
Thomas Edison
Charles Gounod
Henrik Ibsen
Pope Leo XIII
Jules Massenet
Octave Mirabeau
Pope Pius X
Robert Louis
  Stevenson
Jules Verne
Queen Victoria
H. G. Wells
Emile Zola

TWO IMPORTANT
COCAINE BEVERAGES

VIN MARIANI

In 1863, chemist Angelo Mariani patented a mixture of coca extracts and wine as Vin Mariani in the United States. He then introduced his highly concentrated Mariani's Elixir and Mariani Tea onto the market. For advertising purposes, he collected endorsements from the product's most prominent consumers. Thus remarked Fréderic Bartholdi, creator of the Statue of Liberty: *"Vin Mariani seems to brighten, to increase all our faculties; it is very probable that had I taken it twenty years ago, the Statue of Liberty would have attained the height of several hundred meters."*

COCA-COLA

In 1881, pharmacist and war veteran John Styth Pemberton of Atlanta developed a syrup out of wine, kola nuts, damiana, and coca leaf extracts as a remedy for headache, fatigue, and depression: Pemberton's French Wine Coca. When Prohibition came to Atlanta in 1885, Pemberton had to make do without the wine, mixed the syrup with soda water, and subsequently invented Coca-Cola. First sold at pharmacies and in the soda fountains popular at the time, average sales in the beginning totaled only thirteen glasses per day. Needing money to feed his morphine addiction, Pemberton sold the rights and recipe to one-time medical student Asa Griggs Candler for $2,300, eventually making him a very rich man. The only drug left in Coca-Cola since 1906 is caffeine.

THE COPIES: *Velo Cola; Metcalf's Coca Wine; Inca Cola; Café Cola; Dr. Don's Coca; Kola Ade; Kos Kola; Celery Cola; Nicol's Compound Kola Cordial; Kumfort's Cola Extract; Pillsbury's Coke Extract; Vani Cola; Rococola; Quina-Coca; Vin de Coca de Perou; Dr Sampson's Coca Spirits; Sutcliff and Case Company's Beef; Wine and Coca; Lambert Company's Wine of Coca with Peptonate Iron; Maltine's Coca Wine; Liebig's Coca Beef Tonic; Cola-Coca; Dope Cola.*

COCAINE-CONTAINING MEDICATIONS
OF THE NINETEENTH CENTURY

◆ Agnew's Powder ◆ Az-ma-syde ◆
◆ Bernay's Catarrh Cure (Came with a short rubber tube—one end went into the powder, the other into the nostril) ◆
◆ Dr. Tucker's Specific ◆ Nyall's Compound Extract of Damiana ◆
◆ Paine's Celery Compound ◆ Ryno's Hay Fever-'n'-Catarrh Remedy ◆

HOW TO ROLL A JOINT

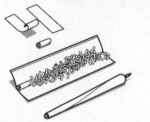

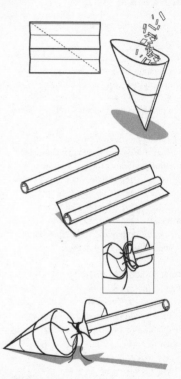

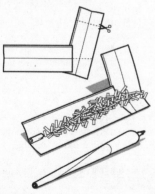

SMALL JOINT

Roll a small, rectangular piece of cardboard into a filter. Distribute the "mix" (marijuana and tobacco) into the paper crease. Roll into a cigarette with the filter at the end, rolling toward the upper end, and lick the adhesive to seal.

LARGE JOINT

Follow the directions for the small joint filter above, then glue a second paper onto the first at a slightly obtuse angle. The objective is to add volume to the front end of the joint. Roll the "mix" in and seal.

TULIP JOINT

Stick two rolling papers together. Form the larger sheet into a funnel or cone shape and glue, then sprinkle the mixture inside. Roll a piece of cardboard into a tube, then roll the tube in another rolling paper and glue. Insert the resulting "stem" into the open side of the funnel, and cinch tightly with string.

BEATLES SONGS

LUCY IN THE SKY WITH DIAMONDS
☞ LSD
"Somebody calls you, you answer quite slowly, a girl with kaleidoscope eyes."

HAPPINESS IS A WARM GUN
☞ HEROIN
"I need a fix 'cause I'm going down."
"When I hold you in my arms and I feel my finger on your trigger, I know nobody can do me no harm."

TOMORROW NEVER KNOWS
☞ LSD
"Turn off your mind, relax and float downstream. It's not dying."

GOT TO GET YOU INTO MY LIFE
☞ MARIJUANA
"I was alone, I took a ride, I didn't know what I would find there. Another road where maybe I could see another kind of mind there."

I AM THE WALRUS
☞ MARIJUANA
"Expert textpert choking smokers."
"Smoke Pot Smoke Pot Everybody Smoke Pot." (Sung by Paul at the end, distorted)

YELLOW SUBMARINE
☞ MARIJUANA
"So we sailed on to the sun, till we found the sea of green."

A DAY IN THE LIFE
☞ MARIJUANA
"Found my way upstairs and had a smoke. Somebody spoke and I went into a dream."

DAY TRIPPER
☞ LSD
"She's a big teaser. She took me half the way there."

DOCTOR ROBERT
☞ AMPHETAMINE
"Take a drink from his special cup."

SHE SAID, SHE SAID
☞ LSD
"I said 'Who put all those things in your head? Things that make me feel that I'm mad.'"

RAIN
☞ MARIJUANA
"Can you hear me, that when it rains and shines, it's just a state of mind?"

STRAWBERRY FIELDS FOREVER
☞ LSD
"But you know I know when it's a dream."

COLD TURKEY
☞ HEROIN
"Thirty-six hours rolling in pain praying to someone free me again." (Solo song by John Lennon, already published in 1969)

CAREER BOOSTS

THROUGH DRUG CONSUMPTION

SIGMUND FREUD

○ After passing his medical exams, the young Dr. Sigmund Freud took a research assistant post at the University of Vienna's Department of Physiology. When the institution refused to promote him even after his third semester, the disappointed Freud gave up hope of becoming a pure researcher and worked as a clinical doctor instead. He began taking cocaine in 1884 as a hedge against despair. On June 2, 1884, he wrote to his bride, Martha Bernays: *"Woe to you, my Princess, when I come. I will kiss you quite red and feed you till you are plump. And if you are forward you shall see who is the stronger, a gentle little girl who doesn't eat enough or a big wild man who has cocaine in his body. In my last severe depression I took coca again and a small dose lifted me to the heights in a wonderful fashion. I am just now busy collecting the literature for a song of praise to this magical substance."* Cocaine gave Freud both the strength and the subject for his 1884 breakthrough essay "On Coca," which catapulted him into international renown. In it, Freud recommends cocaine and other substances as a remedy for physical and mental exhaustion, hypochondria, melancholy, stupor, feelings of fullness, indigestion, belching, and cachexy (emaciation), noting that a dose of only .05 to .10 grams causes *"exhilaration and lasting euphoria, which in no way differs from the normal euphoria of the healthy person. . . . You perceive an increase of self-control and possess more vitality and capacity for work. . . . In other words, you are simply normal, and it is soon hard to believe that you are under the influence of any drug. . . . Long intensive mental or physical work is performed without any fatigue. . . . This result is enjoyed without any of the unpleasant after-effects that follow exhilaration brought about by alcohol. . . . Absolutely no craving for the further use of cocaine appears after the first, or even after repeated taking of the drug; one feels rather a certain curious aversion to it."*

Freud also recommended cocaine in cases of morphine and alcohol withdrawal, fully convinced that the substance was nonaddictive: *"I myself have had occasion to observe a case of rapid withdrawal from morphine under cocaine treatment here, and I saw that a person who had presented the most severe manifestations of collapse at the time of an earlier withdrawal now remained able, with the aid of cocaine, to work and to stay out of bed, and was reminded of his abstinence only by his shivering, diarrhea, and occasionally recurring craving for morphine. He took about 0.40 g of cocaine per day, and by the end of twenty days the morphine abstinence was overcome."*

Reality unfortunately proved his euphoria on cocaine a little premature, but luckily Freud—thanks to the drug's sinister, hallucinogenic side—had already found another, even more resounding topic: dream interpretation and the discovery of the subconscious.

HARRY JACOB ANSLINGER

☼ Anslinger was appointed the first U.S. Commissioner of Narcotic Drugs in 1930 and made a name for himself by sensationalizing marijuana as a rape and murder drug:

"In at least two dozen other comparatively recent cases of murder or degenerate sex attacks, many of them committed by youths, marijuana proved to be a contributing cause. Perhaps you remember the young desperado in Michigan who, a few months ago, caused a reign of terror by his career of burglaries and holdups, finally to be sent to prison for life after kidnapping a Michigan state policeman, killing him, then handcuffing him to the post of a rural mailbox. This young bandit was a marijuana fiend. . . . A sixteen-year-old boy was arrested in California for burglary. Under the influence of marijuana he had stolen a revolver and was on the way to stage a holdup when apprehended. Then there was the nineteen-year-old addict in Columbus, Ohio, who, when police responded to a disturbance complaint, opened fire upon an officer, wounding him three times, and was himself killed by the returning fire of the police. . . "

Defense attorneys across the nation began citing marijuana consumption as grounds for insanity and reduced criminal responsibility. Then, at the end of the 1940s, Anslinger claimed the opposite: that cannabis turned soldiers into pacifists, and Communists were distributing it among American GIs in a plot to undermine U.S. defense readiness.

Anslinger held office until 1962, eventually increasing his staff from 250 to 10,000. In 1961 he celebrated his greatest victory yet: The United Nations Drug Commission passed the Single Convention on Narcotic Drugs, effectively making the War on Drugs the responsibility of each individual country. Anslinger died in 1975—addicted to morphine.

KEN KESEY

☼ In 1959, Ken Kesey signed up as a voluntary participant in LSD experiments at the Menlo Park Veterans Hospital in California. Shortly afterward, he landed a job as a night watchman at the hospital's psychiatric ward. Both experiences inspired his bestseller *One Flew Over the Cuckoo's Nest*. Kesey was arrested for possession of marijuana in 1966 and fled to Mexico before finally serving time in San Francisco. In his old age he complained of *"smokin' holes where my memory used to be."*

ROBBIE WILLIAMS

☼ *"I've really been grappling with depression. It's all linked with my cocaine and ecstasy abuse,"* he said. No other pop star has spoken as candidly about their drug use as Robbie Williams in recent years. When his career hit the skids after being kicked out of the British boy band Take That in 1995, Williams appeared in a 7-Up ad sporting a wig and a beer belly. In Williams's biography, written by British journalist Chris Heath, Williams confesses to taking *"heroin, ecstasy, marijuana, cocaine, alcohol, poppers, speed."* Once he claims to have bought 75,000 euros worth of cocaine. After his song "Angels" became a world success, Williams perfected the trick that would make him the most successful singer in Europe: He had his songs written just a tick above mediocre, then spoke openly about his lack of self-esteem, hunger for attention, and addictions. *"You are going to die. You need to go into rehab now,"* Elton John told him in 1997, when Williams had come to his house to play him some new songs and was *"fucking hammered."* After offering him a drink, John had him carted off to rehab. Williams: *"I started to cry and he started to cry."*

His unrelenting vanity has made him an indispensable character in the European pop scene. Williams's latest voluntary hospitalization happened just in time for his thirty-third birthday on February 13, 2007, though this time the cause was only the antidepressant Seroxat, thirty-six double espressos, and twenty Red Bulls a day. His attitude remains refreshingly ambiguous: *"I hate drugs, I love drugs. As depressing and heartbreaking as it is, as soul-destroying and relationship-destroying as it is, it makes life fucking interesting."*

ANDY WARHOL
☼ The chubby graphic designer (specialty: shoes) from Pittsburgh (1928–1982) took Obetrol (now known as Adderall), a combination of methamphetamines and amphetamines, against drowsiness and weight gain. In the early 1960s he invented Pop Art—speed-fed serialism. Andy Warhol's first paintings are of everyday objects and commercial products like the well-known Campbell's soup cans; he later simplified and accelerated the process with silkscreen. His studio, which he called the Factory, was populated with junkies, strippers, and transvestites in the sixties, and cocainists in suits in the seventies. One of his trademark aphorisms was *"I think everybody should be a machine."* Jackson Pollock, fifties figurehead of the heterosexual, alcohol-soaked, strongman art that Warhol both loathed and envied, had said, *"I am nature."*

Warhol was a so-called narcovoyeur who loved experiencing people at their absolute limit. *"I wonder if Edie will commit suicide,"* he mused about Edie Sedgwick, who by then had slipped from speed to heroin and from Factory-superstar fame to near oblivion. *"I hope she lets me know so I can film it."* Sedgwick was found dead in her mother's swimming pool. Later, Warhol enjoyed observing his cocaine- and

HORSE ON COKE

In his book *The Murderers* (1961), American antidrug advocate Harry Anslinger writes about a racehorse doped with a so-called shotgun: fourteen parts cocaine, three parts heroin and other stimulants. The horse was so agitated that five men needed to hold it down. It won the race but bucked the rider shortly after leaving the gate. His owner was trampled to death after attempting to discipline the horse with a club.

Quaalude-fueled entourage at Studio 54 (though he considered selling the pills given to him instead of taking them). His last stimulating kick was the creative rejuvenation with the help of heroin-addicted painter Jean-Michel Basquiat.

KATE MOSS

◌ "I don't do any more drugs than anybody else. Not class A, especially heroin, after what happened to Davide," the supermodel said, referring to Davide Sorrenti, a fashion photographer who died of an overdose and whose brother Mario was Moss's longtime boyfriend. Kate Moss checked into the Priory Hospital as early as 1998 to treat her addiction, explaining afterward that "almost everyone I know does drugs. What am I supposed to do? Be like Bill Clinton and say, 'I didn't inhale'? Like when he said, 'I didn't have sex with that woman. She just sucked me off.'" Two years later she also admitted that fashion industry boredom had driven her to drug use as a means of escape.

Scandal ensued in September 2005 when the British Mirror printed photographs of the model snorting cocaine in a recording studio. The photos—and her apparently ruinous affair with Pete Doherty—cost the model several top contracts, including those with H&M and Burberry. Just a few months and one Meadows stay later, she was back on the cover of the world's most influential magazines (among them Vanity Fair and W) and signing even more lucrative deals than before. Her income in 2006 was reportedly three times what it had been the previous year; Moss's agency counted 150 companies eager to hire her for their ad campaigns.

In the summer of 2006, the Sun reported that Moss had snorted cocaine during a visit to Nelson Mandela's home several years before. A modeling agent present at the time recalled, "She was insatiable." Experts analyzed recent photos for cocaine-related damage to the nasal cavity (so-called saddle nose), as evidenced by a slightly collapsed nose tip. Moss separated from Pete Doherty in the summer of 2007.

JÖRG IMMENDORFF

◌ The famed German painter Jörg Immendorff (1945–2007) was celebrated for his gigantic canvases in the 1980s, then slipped into relative obscurity before developing Lou Gehrig's disease in 1997. Cocaine and whores were a source of comfort to the artist as he was dealing with the increasingly debilitating, fatal neurodegenerative illness.

In August 2003, six policemen, three district attorneys, and a sniffer dog burst into his luxury suite at the Steigenberger Hotel in Düsseldorf, finding him in possession of several grams of cocaine. In a media-savvy move, he was also surrounded by seven prostitutes—with two more on the way. Immendorff, who apologetically excused the behavior by pointing to his "orientalism," was sentenced to eleven months on probation and fined 150,000 euros. Just two days after the media storm surrounding Immendorff's immaculately staged orgy, people received the invitation to his retrospective Aualand. The Bild newspaper hired the artist to illustrate its edition of the Bible, and a comprehensive solo exhibition of his work opened in 2005 at the Neue Nationalgalerie in Berlin.

SELF-REFLECTIONS: THE BEST OF

KEITH RICHARDS

"I've never turned blue in somebody else's bathroom. I consider that the height of bad manners."

"People talk about cocaine addiction all the time, but I know what addiction is: opium, heroin, you know? Cocaine is just a bad habit."

"The only recurring dreams I can remember are all on cold turkey, and it was always that the dope was hidden behind the wallpaper. And in the morning, you'd wake up and see fingernail marks where you actually tried to do something about it."

"The strangest thing I've tried to snort? My father. I snorted my father. He was cremated and I couldn't resist grinding him up with a little bit of blow. My dad wouldn't have cared, he didn't give a shit. It went down pretty well, and I'm still alive."

"I was number one on the Who's Likely to Die list for ten years. I mean, I was really disappointed when I fell off the list."

"Cold turkey is not so bad after you've done it ten or twelve times."

FRIEND NUMBER 16

Robin Williams

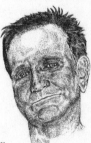

"Cocaine for me was a place to hide. Most people get hyper on coke. It slowed me down. Sometimes it made me paranoid and impotent, but mostly it just made me withdrawn," says the actor with the trademark, sometimes hard-to-bear hyperness. Maybe his early fame as Mork from Ork was too much for him. Comedian Robin Williams (born 1951) occasionally admitted taking massive amounts of cocaine in the seventies and was with fellow comedian John Belushi on the night he died of an overdose. At a New Year's Eve party hosted by Woody Allen, Williams reportedly demanded to know who the fat guy sitting next to him was, referring to Robert De Niro, who had put on weight for his role in *Raging Bull*. Afterward Williams peed in a Ming vase and was kicked out. He apparently kicked his drug habit after becoming a father. In the summer of 2006, a representative announced that Williams was in treatment for a drinking problem after twenty years of sobriety. There was no mention of cocaine. He is credited with the famous one-liner: "Cocaine is God's way of saying you're making too much money."

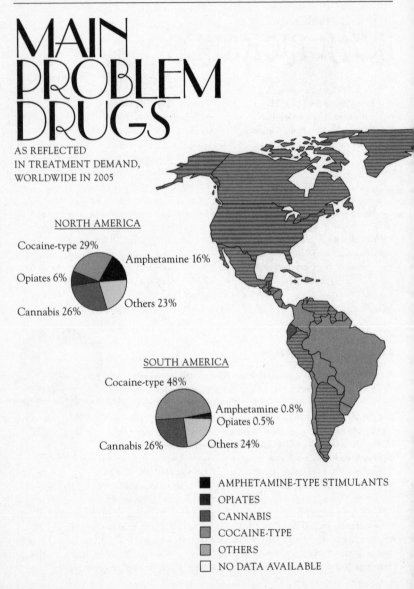

INGO NIERMANN AND ADRIANO SACK

MAIN PROBLEM DRUGS

AS REFLECTED
IN TREATMENT DEMAND,
WORLDWIDE IN 2005

NORTH AMERICA

Cocaine-type 29%

Amphetamine 16%

Opiates 6%

Others 23%

Cannabis 26%

SOUTH AMERICA

Cocaine-type 48%

Amphetamine 0.8%
Opiates 0.5%

Cannabis 26%

Others 24%

- AMPHETAMINE-TYPE STIMULANTS
- OPIATES
- CANNABIS
- COCAINE-TYPE
- OTHERS
- NO DATA AVAILABLE

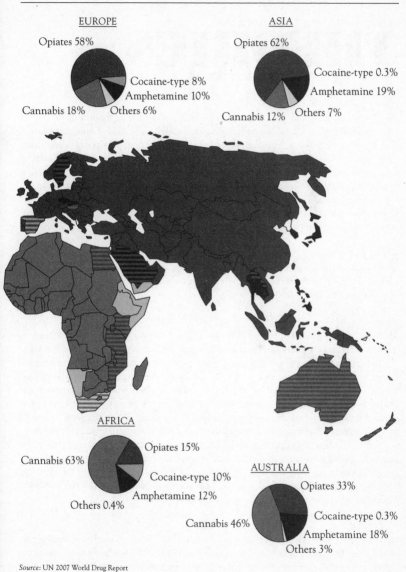

EUROPE
Opiates 58%
Cocaine-type 8%
Amphetamine 10%
Cannabis 18%   Others 6%

ASIA
Opiates 62%
Cocaine-type 0.3%
Amphetamine 19%
Cannabis 12%   Others 7%

AFRICA
Opiates 15%
Cannabis 63%
Cocaine-type 10%
Amphetamine 12%
Others 0.4%

AUSTRALIA
Opiates 33%
Cocaine-type 0.3%
Amphetamine 18%
Cannabis 46%
Others 3%

Source: UN 2007 World Drug Report

IMPORTANT AND NOT-SO-IMPORTANT

THEORIES

DEVELOPED UNDER THE INFLUENCE OF DRUGS

MEDITATIONS

✱ The Roman emperor Marcus Aurelius (121–180) was more of a philosopher than a military leader. His *Meditations*, still widely read today, are a bid for stoic equanimity. He himself was partial to regular doses of opium. His personal physician Galen wrote: *"We know of Marcus Aurelius that he immunized himself daily with an amount the size of an Egyptian bean, swallowing it down without water or mixing it with wine or something similar. When this resulted in his nodding off while going about his daily business, he left out the poppy juice. This had the consequence however, because of his previous habit, that he lay awake for the large part of the night unable to sleep...for this reason he felt forced to take the opium-containing liquid once more."*

NEOPLATONISM

✱ The Greek philosopher Plotinus (205–270) regularly used opium. The very elastic understanding of space in his emanation doctrine could easily be attributed to a reality perceived during opium intoxication.

THE DOCTRINE OF STHENIC AND ASTHENIC DISEASES

✱ The Scottish physician Dr. John Brown (1735–1788) claimed that life itself was a certain reservoir of "excitability"; every day it is depleted a little more until one day we die. For Brown there were only two kinds of diseases, sthenic and asthenic, and two remedies: opium and alcohol. Sthenic disease was caused by an overstimulation of the senses for which a sedative—alcohol—was the only cure; asthenic illness was due to understimulation and could be helped by opium. This pleasingly simple theory and treatment plan enjoyed enormous popularity in Europe until the beginning of the nineteenth century and in American alternative medicine all the way into the twentieth century. Brown himself suffered from severe depression and died as a consequence of high alcohol and opium consumption. Opium is generally classified as a sedative and not as a stimulant; Brown begged to differ, pointing to how it was given to Turkish soldiers to improve their combat effectiveness. What Brown didn't know: The soldiers were not doped with the substance before the fight; they received it afterward as a reward.

ASTHENICISM

✱ The German Romantics were also firm believers in John Brown's theory. Brown reasoned that 97% of all diseases were asthenic and only 3% sthenic. Novalis, who also suffered from the "asthenic disease" tuberculosis, saw asthetics as capable of attaining a more conscientious and therefore higher level of life. External stimuli must be reduced or blunted as much as possible to increase internal stimulation, thus shifting the mind-body balance at the body's expense. Opium was a source of comfort for Novalis, and using it was a means of producing new internal stimuli. In 1798 he wrote, *"What shall restore me when hopeless and queasy, but bitter almond water and opium."* One year later he rhymed in his "Hymns to the Night": *"What springs up all at once so sweetly boding in my heart, and stills the soft air of sadness? Dost thou also take a pleasure in us, dark Night? What holdest thou under thy mantle, that with hidden power affects my soul? Precious balm drips from thy hand out of its bundle of poppies."*

PSYCHOANALYSIS
✻ Sigmund Freud had already been sworn off cocaine for ten years by the time his central work, *The Interpretation of Dreams*, was published in 1900. But the idea that dreams show people their own symbolically encrypted fantasy worlds and that they can be deciphered in therapeutic conversation owes a great deal to cocaine. This is not only because of cocaine's lowering of psychic inhibitions; it also lends the necessary meaning to whatever cockamamie ideas arise in the process.

NATIONAL SOCIALISM
✻ In his book *Spear of Destiny* (1973), author Trevor Ravenscroft traces Hitler's national socialist visions to peyote taken in Vienna before World War I. The peyote was all the more potent on account of Hitler's fasting at the time.

THE THEORY OF MASS RETRIBUTION
✻ Because of his open speculation that the United States could bear 20 million atomic deaths, the nuclear deterrence theorist Herman Kahn (1922–1983) inspired the Stanley Kubrick character Dr. Strangelove. Yet the more than three-hundred-pound Kahn also nursed a shy love of hippies, met with radical left student leader Abbie Hoffman, and repeatedly took LSD. Timothy Leary speculated that it was LSD that enabled Kahn's clear-eyed contemplation of atomic warfare.

ATWA = AIR-TREES-WATER-ANIMALS OR ALL THE WAY ALIVE
✻ Fresh out of prison in the 1960s, Charles Manson (born 1934) founded a paranoid cult supported by numerous LSD trips. *"Paranoia is just a kind of awareness,"* he explained in an interview with *Rolling Stone*. *"Have you ever seen the coyote in the desert? Watching, tuned in, completely aware. Christ on the cross, the coyote in the desert—it's the same thing, man. The coyote is beautiful. You learn from the coyote just like you can learn from a child. A baby is born into this world into a state of fear. Total paranoia and awareness."* Manson fuelled fear and persecution anxiety among his followers in their commune, and declared the reversal of all values: God is Satan, Hitler Christ, Death Life. For Manson, all violence was permissible as long as it was in the service of ATWA, the all-encompassing life

principle. Leading his "family" into a "holy war," they attacked and brutally murdered several people—among others, the actress Sharon Tate—and waited for the Armed SS to return from outer space. He rehearsed a desert war with an armada of stolen dune buggies, trying to imitate the tactics of Nazi field marshal "Desert Fox" Rommel. Manson followers said that he could bring dead birds and horses back to life. When a girl giving him fellatio allegedly became so aroused that she bit off his penis, he used mental powers to reattach it. All five eyewitnesses were under the influence of LSD.

PANDROGYNITY
❊ By the end of the 1980s Genesis P. Orridge (born 1950), cofounder of the industrial rock band Throbbing Gristle, only crawled across the stage at concerts, completely hidden from view. The only thing the audience could make out through the thick dry-ice haze were the letters LSD, spelled out in lights on his baseball cap. Today P. Orridge has once again reemerged—as a hermaphrodite with breast implants, gold teeth, collagen lips, and tightened skin. S/he believes that humankind's only chance at peace and happiness lies in its ability to unite the masculine and feminine within.

WAYS TO GET HIGH WITH
NO DRUGS AT ALL

✳ FASTING—The faster will notice significant body odor and bad breath after a few days, but soon feels pleasantly light and at times euphoric. Those who continue to fast may also become delirious; many medieval saints owed their visions to excessive fasting and famine-induced malnutrition.

✳ LUCID DREAMING—In a lucid dream (from Latin, *lux*, meaning "light") the sleeper is conscious of the fact that he or she is dreaming. Tibetan monks, yogis, and Indian shamans have been cultivating this art for centuries. Today, psychophysiologist Stephen LaBerge (born 1947) is a leading lucid dream researcher. His specially developed

DreamLight is a sleeping mask that sends light signals to the eyelids as soon as the wearer enters a dream phase. The signal seen in the dream can be recognized as a sign that he or she is dreaming.

✳ RUNNER'S HIGH—A sudden burst of euphoria after approximately sixty minutes of running, also attributed to endorphin release.

✳ SEX—Significantly faster than jogging, sex releases endorphins in a mere matter of minutes.

✳ SUICIDE—Brain autopsies of suicide victims have shown extremely high endorphin levels.

✳ TREPANATION—In 1965, Dutchman Bart Hughes drilled a hole in the roof of his own skull in order to reduce the pressure in his head and permanently raise the volume of blood in his brain. Hughes remarked after the operation: "*I think that no adult organization can work optimally unless each adult in the organization has been trepanned.*"

✳ SPIN AROUND FAST IN A CIRCLE —Works not only for children. Sufi dervishes also whirl themselves like a top into a trance.

✳ FLAGELLATION—People disposed to masochism take pleasure in causing themselves pain. Anyone else would have to take it to such an excruciating extreme that the body counteracts by releasing large amounts of endorphins, hormones similar to opiates. One particularly effective way to inflict huge amounts of pain on oneself is self-flagellation, also called self-whipping. This was a common way to do penance in the Middle Ages. The pope damned the practice as heretical in 1349; flagellators were suspected of deriving an all-too-physical ecstasy from the whip. An extreme example of this is the nun Wilbirgis, who in 1248 sequestered herself in a cell at the St. Florian monastery in Austria. Her confessor Einwik wrote: "*As Wilbirgis entered the service of God, she fortified herself against temptations with extreme physical mortification. For in those days she enclosed herself in an iron shackle so designed, that she could tighten and loosen it at will. Then she was of the thought that she would for once like to loosen it not out of necessity, but because she wished to; and so had it attached to her in such a way that it could no longer be loosened at all, even if she wanted to. After wearing this for two years, her flesh began to fester beneath it. Puss began to spill over it, the raw flesh swelled over it; the ring itself was completely hidden from view. After another two years had passed, however, it broke away in four pieces, painfully ripping away much of the rotted flesh with it.*"

✳ HEADSTAND—In the sixties it was popular to spend long periods of time in a headstand, even in company, as a way of increasing blood flow to the brain. The "high" experienced is touted by head-standers as the natural state, because—or so it is assumed—a person's blood circulation is still that of a four-legged animal and is not up to the constant standing and sitting. The occasional headstand can replace a caffeine or nicotine kick. Beginners are advised to support the majority of their bodyweight with their arms.

✳ HYPERVENTILATION—Quick or heavy breathing leads to a surplus of fresh air in the lungs. Though the blood's oxygen concentration is barely affected, the increased exhalation of carbon dioxide from the body raises the blood pH, making it more basic and reducing the number of free calcium ions. Calcium deficiency can lead to cramps, prickles, and twitching, but can also induce a trance. Psychologist Dr. Stanislav Graof leads workshops in holotropic breathing—nothing but hyperventilation with meditation music and pillows.

ALLEGED MAXIMUM DOSES SURVIVED

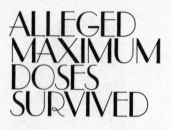

CAFFEINE

⁝ No known lethal case to date, though the writer Honoré de Balzac is sometimes said to have died of caffeine poisoning. In his final days he drank an average of approximately fifty cups of strong black coffee every day, sometimes eighty. He suffered choking spells, dropsy, and the early stages of blindness; his face turned purple, he wheezed, and could speak only in fits and starts. His legs swelled up, and he had abscesses and open wounds. In the end he could only groan.

ECSTASY

⁝ Doctors at the St. George's Medical School in London reported a patient in April 2006 who swallowed up to twenty-five ecstasy pills a day, about 40,000 pills in all. Seven years later, the thirty-seven-year-old complained of a spotty memory, hallucinations, and depression, and his neck and jaw muscles were so tight that he often couldn't open his mouth.

CANNABIS

⁝ To this day not one death has been directly attributed to cannabis consumption. Laboratory tests with rhesus apes have established the deadly dose as an intravenous dose of 128 milligrams per bodyweight kilogram before apnea and heart failure set in. For a 170- to 180-pound man that would be—assuming the results can be transferred to humans—around .35 ounce of pure active ingredient, or 7 ounces of marijuana.

COCAINE

⁝ Just 1 to 2 grams at a time (either snorted or injected) can be lethal, though fatalities have also been reported at much lower doses. The body can handle a much bigger dose of the substance if smoked in its freebase form. The Peruvian doctor Raoul Jeri claims to have watched one study participant smoke 50 grams of coca paste in a single sitting.

LSD

⁝ Is effective in doses of .02–.1 milligram, but 20 milligrams have been survived—by one LSD dealer who swallowed it during a police search. He suffered extreme psychosis, which faded after thirteen days, with no apparent aftereffects. There have been no known LSD fatalities to date, though in rare cases taking it has lead to situations with deadly consequences (such as jumping out of a window). German cabaret artist Wolfgang Neuss claimed of himself: "*In seven years I have taken 6,000 LSD trips. I'm hoping to be renewed.*"

FRIEND NUMBER 17
Donatella Versace

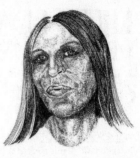

"I was always afraid of what I would discover if I looked too deep in myself," said fashion designer Donatella Versace (born 1955) of her recovery from cocaine addiction. After trying the drug for the first time at the age of thirty-two, she remained addicted for eighteen years. *"I had so much fun. I had the best time of my life,"* she said. When her brother Gianni was shot dead outside of his Miami Beach villa, she took over creative direction of the company. Versace tried to stop her substance abuse habit but soon found herself mixing cocaine with sedatives, then fighting her chronic headaches with *"lots of Excedrin."* In February 2004, Versace collapsed after a fashion show: *"I was crying, laughing, crying, sleeping. People couldn't understand me. I screamed, I slept. Not even I understood what I was saying."* Her hair was falling out and she lost weight. Elton John, tireless helper to addicts in need, convinced her to join a rehabilitation program. She then flew to the desert, where she encountered *"spirituality, beauty, and even glamour."* Writing about her 2006 summer collection fashion critic Suzy Menkes compared the pieces to the earlier, more flamboyant designs: *"The Versace girl now has a life before the happy hour."* A year later Versace publicly stated that her daughter Allegra, heiress to the fashion house, had long suffered from anorexia and was seeking professional help.

REGISTERED DRUG USERS IN
Kazakhstan, Kyrgyzstan, Tajikistan, and Uzbekistan

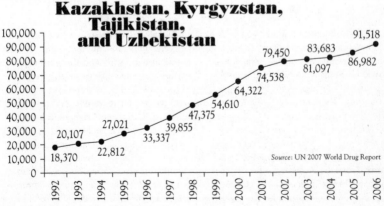

Source: UN 2007 World Drug Report

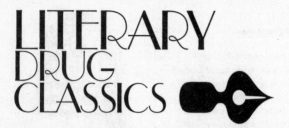

LITERARY DRUG CLASSICS

ALICE'S ADVENTURES IN WONDERLAND (1865) BY LEWIS CARROLL

●◆ The title heroine escapes from a boring picnic by following a rabbit down his hole and finds herself in a puzzling new world. Among other characters, Alice meets a caterpillar sitting on a very large mushroom. A bite from one side of the mushroom causes the consumer to grow; a bite from the other makes her shrink. The author himself enjoyed drinking laudanum.

THE STRANGE CASE OF DR. JEKYLL AND MR. HYDE (1886)
BY ROBERT LOUIS STEVENSON

●◆ Stevenson wrote the book on cocaine and managed to pen the 60,000 words, including two complete revisions, in only six days. The description of good Jekyll's metamorphosis into the scurrilous Hyde bears a striking resemblance to an insipient cocaine high: *"There was something strange in my sensations, something indescribably new and, from its very novelty, incredibly sweet. I felt younger, lighter, happier in body; within I was conscious of a heady recklessness, a current of disordered sensual images running like a millrace in my fancy, a solution of the bonds of obligation, an unknown but not an innocent freedom of the soul."*

COCAINE (1918) BY WALTER RHEINER

●◆ Berlin, just after World War I: The cocainist Tobias effortlessly buys the substance from his local pharmacy; one hexagonal bottle is enough for several sips or injections. In the last night before his suicide, Tobias hallucinates a giant whip cracking and snapping over his head. Walter Rheiner himself died of a morphine overdose in a sleazy Berlin hotel in 1925. When World War I began, he and Johannes R. Becher (who later wrote the German Democratic Republic national anthem) tried to escape active military duty by taking massive amounts of drugs—to no avail—and Rheiner never shook the cocaine addiction.

STEPPENWOLF (1927) BY HERMANN HESSE

●◆ *"Don't dream it. Be it."* pretty much sums up the essence of this young adult literary classic. Harry "Steppenwolf" Haller—like his author, fifty years old—wanders aimlessly through a small town where he keeps seeing a sign that reads "MAGIC THEATER—

ENTRANCE NOT FOR EVERYBODY—FOR MADMEN ONLY." But Harry Haller prefers to drink wine at a pub called the Steel Helmet before he, finally, four-fifths into the book, enters the magic theater. There he smokes a long, thin, yellow cigarette with smoke *"as thick as incense,"* and *"slowly sips"* a sweet herbal liquid: *"Its effect was immeasurably enlivening and delightful—as though one were filled with gas and had become weightless."* He takes a look in the mirror, learns to laugh at himself, and dissociates into several different egos. He then climbs into one of the theater's several loges and learns how to shoot down at wealthy peoples' automobiles. He has a vile taste of chocolate and blood in his mouth. He is fifteen again and happily falls back in love with his old childhood sweethearts. He meets Mozart at a performance of *Don Giovanni*; Mozart tells him, *"You see, it works all right without the saxophone."* Brahms and Wagner are forced to repent for their bombastic music. Mozart switches on an old radio, incensing Haller. But with Mozart's help, Haller learns to love its *"unappetizing tone-slime,"* because *"all of life is like that."* Haller grabs Mozart's pigtail, is flung through the universe, and wakes up again.

JUNKIE (1953) BY WILLIAM S. BURROUGHS

●◆ The book tells the story of Burroughs's own opium and heroin dependency. At first he gets the substance by prescription, but the drug laws in postwar America soon become significantly tougher. Police officers on the streets force suspicious-looking passersby to show their forearms; anyone with track marks is immediately sent to jail. Burroughs starts robbing drunks and vagrants to pay for his addiction, then switches to small-time dealing. He is arrested several times, keeps moving to one city after another, and makes countless attempts at rehabilitation. But for Burroughs, rehab is at the outset just another addictive episode: *"I wasn't high on the hop; I was high on withdrawal tone-up. Junk is an inoculation of death that keeps the body in a condition of emergency. When the junky is cut off, emergency reactions continue. Sensations sharpen, the addict is aware of his visceral processes to an uncomfortable degree, peristalsis and secretion go unchecked. No matter what his actual age, the kicking addict is liable to the emotional excesses of a child or an adolescent."* Unlike many a stereotypical drug memoir, this book doesn't end in remorse. Burroughs writes, *"I think I am in better health now as a result of using junk at intervals than I would be if I had never been an addict. When you stop growing you start dying. An addict never stops growing."*

ON THE ROAD (1957) BY JACK KEROUAC

●◆ Typed on an endless roll, constantly on speed—though the best thing about the book is its description of speed's effects: *"He rubbed his jaw furiously, he swung the car and passed three trucks, he roared into downtown Testament, looking in every direction and seeing everything in an arc of 180 degrees around his eyeballs without moving his head. Bang, he found a parking space in no time, and we were parked. He leaped out of the car. (. . .) He had become absolutely mad in his movements; he seemed to be doing everything at the same time. It was a shaking of the head, up and down, side-*

ways; jerky, vigorous hands; quick walking, sitting, crossing the legs, uncrossing, getting up, rubbing the hands, rubbing his fly, hitching his pants, looking up and saying 'Am,' and sudden slitting of the eyes to see everywhere; and all the time he was grabbing me by the ribs and talking, talking."

THE THREE STIGMATA OF PALMER ELDRITCH (1965) BY PHILIP K. DICK

●❖ All of Philip K. Dick's (1928–1982) science fiction, from his first book in the 1950s on, was written on speed. His biographer Emmanuel Carrère estimates that he consumed up to one thousand tablets per week. Unable to quit taking the pills despite life-threatening liver cirrhosis, his then girlfriend checked him into a psychiatric hospital. According to Dick, the doctors released him soon afterward, stating that the speed had no physical effect on him because it wouldn't reach the neural epithelium—his liver was already too damaged. He would have had to inject the amphetamine for it to have any effect at all. Finally Dick pulled himself together and for once managed to write a novel—*A Scanner Darkly*—without speed, claiming that it felt just the same as before. This was Philip K. Dick's greatest fear: finding himself in a world where he no longer had to take drugs to feel like he was on them. And his great question: Is this world for real or am I crazy? It's too late to ask questions in *Palmer Eldritch*. The new drug Chew-Z seduces the user into a penurious world where he is constantly running into a steely-toothed creature—Palmer Eldritch. Days later, just when the user thinks his horror trip is over, his typical surroundings turn to dust and Palmer Eldritch appears once more. Finally the user himself turns into Palmer Eldritch. Philip K. Dick was so spooked by the novel that he could never read it again. For several weeks he saw Palmer Eldritch in the clouds—pure evil—chaos, absolute entropy.

CARCINOMA ANGELS (1967) BY NORMAN SPINRAD

●❖ A multibillionaire dying of cancer takes a drug cocktail consisting of the stimulant Benzedrine, various hallucinogens, morphine (to kill the pain), vlut (a Tibetan poison that causes temporary blindness), and tympanoline (which temporarily deadens the auditory nerves). Deprived of all sensory stimulation, all alone and alert in his fantastic thoughts, he manages to project himself into his own bloodstream. There he meets the Carcinoma Angels—on black motorcycles, black dragons, and fighter planes—and destroys them with machine guns, light sabers, and antiaircraft fire. The multibillionaire triumphs over cancer and lands in a psychiatric hospital.

THE TEACHINGS OF DON JUAN (1968) BY CARLOS CASTANEDA

●❖ Carlos, a California anthropology student, meets the old Mexican Indian Don Juan in Arizona in 1960 and is introduced to the magical powers of the peyote cactus. The bitter taste of the tubers makes him nauseous; his stomach cramping, he falls to the floor and asks Don Juan for water. All of a sudden a dog approaches and starts drinking it. He tries to chase it away but when the animal suddenly becomes transparent, Carlos sees how the water flows through the dog, luminous, and shoots out through its hairs.

Carlos leans over and starts drinking from the water dish with him: ". . . and as I drank, I saw the fluid running through my veins setting up hues of red and yellow and green. I drank more and more. I drank until I was all afire; I was all aglow." Soon afterward, he and the dog are running off together "toward a yellow warmth that came from some indefinite place. And there we played. We played and wrestled until I knew his wishes and he knew mine. (. . .) I could make him move his legs by twisting my toes, and every time he nodded his head I felt an irresistible impulse to jump. But his most impish act was to make me scratch my head with my foot while I sat; he did it by flapping his ears from side to side. This action was to me utterly, unbearably funny. Such a touch of grace and irony; such mastery, I thought (. . .) I had forgotten that I was a man! The sadness of such an irreconcilable situation was so intense that I wept."

Don Juan seems confident. The peyote appears to have "accepted" Carlos. The dog was none other than the peyote itself, playing with him. Even though Carlos vomited, it was "only ten times."

THE RULES OF ATTRACTION (1987) BY BRET EASTON ELLIS
●◆ The American author's second novel is about a few students who spend their nights having sex and doing drugs. The book follows the different protagonists' perspectives, which at times show very diverging perceptions of the same circumstances. Drugs are consumed indiscriminately—mostly cannabis, cocaine, alcohol, and ecstasy. One of the kids is astonished when he unintentionally has sex without the influence of drugs.

FRISK (1991) BY DENNIS COOPER
●◆ In Part I of the American writer's series of books on sexual desire and sadistic fantasies, drugs are the least of what the reader is faced with. His works are flinty-eyed, maniacal protocols: "I pushed in my cock. I couldn't fit much inside. The difference was too great. When I forced it he started to squeal. So the Germans rushed up with a long piece of rope and tied the kid's hands in case he decided to struggle, though like I said, Dutch guys don't fight back. Period. Physically anyway. Ferdinand got out the heroin and cooked it up in a spoon. He shot it into a vein behind one of the kid's knees. It took effect right away. The kid's squeals sort of faded. He sounded more like a cat mewing."

A MILLION LITTLE PIECES (2003) BY JAMES FREY
●◆ Former crackhead and alcoholic James Frey's memoir was celebrated as both an unsparing self-help book and literary triumph in equal parts when the Oprah Winfrey Show catapulted it onto the bestseller list. That is, until parts of the professed factual account turned out to be fiction. This does nothing to diminish the intensity of the first two hundred pages, in particular: With four missing teeth, a broken nose, and a hole in his cheek, the narrator's parents check him into a treatment center, where he encounters drug fantasies, fellow patients, and, of course, love. His formidable drug career

is described in the third person and not without pride: *"Two arrests at eighteen. First overdose, first case of alcohol poisoning. Tried to quit again, lasted two days. Vomited blood for the first time, had first cocaine-induced bloody nose. Nineteen. Blacked out five days a week, vomited five days a week. Pissed bed for the first time. Shook visibly when not drinking. Woke up for the first time without knowing where he was or how he got there. Twenty. Blacked out seven days a week. Vomited several times a day, seven days a week. Smoked cocaine for the first time, smoked methamphetamine for the first time, smoked PCP for the first time."*

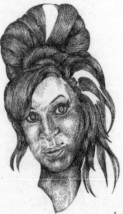

FRIEND NUMBER 18
Amy Winehouse

"She requires special treatment to continue her ongoing recovery from drug addiction," her record label Universal declared in January 2008—an unusually but unavoidably frank statement given the singer/songwriter from England's very public struggle with apparently any available drug. Amy Winehouse (born 1983) released her hit album *Back to Black* in 2006 including the oddly prophetic—or maybe just utterly personal—song "Rehab": *"They tried to make me go to rehab, but I said no, no, no."*

Though her distinctive voice and outrageous beehive hairdo had propelled her into the limelight even before that, it was the singer's sophisticated old-school soul album and rapidly worsening lifestyle that made her one of pop culture's most promising newcomers and tabloid stars of 2007.

Photos of her husband Blake Fielder-Civil and herself with deep scratches on their faces were published in August, and both entered a rehab clinic but left after a couple of days. She was arrested for marijuana possession in Norway, walked the streets only wearing a signal red bra, at some point one tooth was visibly missing, and she bleached her signature black hair blond. In January 2008 she was filmed smoking crack and talking about having taken ecstasy and Valium.

Unlike Britney Spears, another celebrity fighting her own very personal war on drugs (or not?), Winehouse belongs to the group of exceptionally gifted musicians who, through their struggles seems to achieve even higher artistic levels. Both Prince and George Michael declared themselves "fans" of the troubled star and have expressed a desire to work with her.

Ironically she has also made a strong contribution to the perception of drug problems as being part of contemporary entertainment. In summer 2007, girls were spotted wearing T-shirts with the slogan "Rehab Is the New Black."

Hallucinations

OCCURRING WHEN COCAINE IS TAKEN FREQUENTLY
OR IN HIGH DOSES

- OLFACTORY HALLUCINATIONS: odor of smoke, gasoline, feces, urine, gas
- HYPERACUSIS: heightened sense of hearing
- TIME LAPSE AND TIME EXPANSION
- POLYOPSIA: "seeing double" or in multiples
- DYSMORPHOSIS: objects change shape
- "SNOW LIGHTS" WHEN THE EYES ARE CLOSED: light reflections

- MICROPSIA: objects appear much smaller than they are
- MACROPSIA: objects appear much larger than they are
- ZOOPSIA: hallucination of small, rapidly moving animals, such as white lice with red eyes or flying worms
- TACTILE HALLUCINATIONS: bacteria, worms, mites, fleas, glass splinters, sand, tiny crystals, spiders, and snakes on and underneath the skin, including the mucous membranes (the tongue, for example)

ILLEGAL DRUG USE WORLDWIDE

Total world population: 6,475 billion

World population age fifteen to sixty-four: 4,177 billion

Annual prevalence of drug use: 200 million people (4.8%)

Monthly prevalence of drug use: 110 million people (2.6%)

Source: UN 2007 World Drug Report

Problem drug use: 25 million people (0.6%)

COCAINE SONGS

1927 "*Dope Head Blues*" Victoria Spivey
"*Cocaine Blues*" (I) Luke Jordan

1930-1933
"*Cocaine Habit Blues*" Memphis Jug Band
"*Minnie the Moocher*" Cab Calloway
"*Minnie the Moocher's Wedding Day*" Cab Calloway
"*Kickin' the Gong Around*" Cab Calloway

1934 "*Take a Whiff on Me*" (I) Huddie Ledbetter

1938 "*I Get a Kick out of You*" Cole Porter
"*Wacky Dust*" Ella Fitzgerald

1941-1957 "*Stuff Stomp*" Elijah Jones
"*Juncker Blues*" Champion Jack Dupree
"*Cocaine Blues*" (II) Slumber Nichols' Western Aces

1964 "*Cocaine Blues*" (III) Reverend Gary Davis
"*Cocaine Done Killed My Baby*" Mance Lipscomb

1966 "*Think Twice*" Jackie Wilson & LaVern Baker
"*New Amphetamine Shriek*" The Fugs

1967 "*Poverty Train*" Laura Nyro
"*Snow White*" Winston's Fumbs

1968 "*Memo from Turner*" Mick Jagger
"*Amphetamine Annie*" Canned Heat

1969 "*Substitute*" The Who
"*Let It Bleed*" Rolling Stones
"*Sister Morphine*" (I) Marianne Faithfull

1970 "*Cocaine Katy*" Moloch
"*Mau Mau*" Jefferson Starship
"*Draggin' the Line*" Tommy James

1971 "*Sweet Cocaine*" Fred Neil
"*Hi Jack*" Jefferson Starship
"*Have a Whiff of Me*" Mungo Jerry
"*Take a Whiff on Me*" (II) The Byrds
"*Earth Mother*" Paul Kantner & Grace Slick
"*Casey Jones*" Grateful Dead
"*Moonlight Mile*" Rolling Stones
"*Snowblind Friend*" Steppenwolf
"*Can't You Hear Me Knockin'?*" Rolling Stones
"*Truckin'*" Grateful Dead
"*Sister Morphine*" (II) Rolling Stones
"*Cocaine*" (I) Andwella's Dream
"*I Found Out*" John Lennon
"*Short Dogs and Englishmen*" Pacific Gas & Electric

1972 "Pusherman" Curtis Mayfield
"No Thing on Me (Cocaine Song)" Curtis Mayfield
"All Down the Line" Rolling Stones
"Mr. Charlie" Grateful Dead
"Sailin' Shoes" Little Feat
"Willin'" Little Feat

1973 "Dealer's Blues" Doug Sahm and Band
"The Cover of Rolling Stone" Dr. Hook & the Medicine Show
"Let It Roar Like a Flood" Larry Estridge
"Troubleshooter" Larry Estridge
"Lonesome L.A. Cowboy" New Riders of the Purple Sage

1974 "Sailing Shoes" Robert Palmer   "Guilty" (I) Joe Cocker
"Cocaine Blues" (IV) The Sharks
"Cocaine Carolina" Johnny Cash

1975 "Guilty" (II) Nazareth
"No No Song" Hoyt Axton

1976 "Life in the Fast Lane" The Eagles
"Cocaine in My Brain" Dillinger
"Station to Station" David Bowie
"Snowblind" Black Sabbath

1977 "Ain't Nobody's Business" Taj Mahal
"Snowblind Friend" Hoyt Axton
"Dandy in the Underworld" Marc Bolan & T. Rex
"Nothing but Time" Jackson Browne
"Mr. Jones" Steve Gibbons Band
"Nite City" Nite City
"Nightclubbing" Iggy Pop

1978 "Tequila Is Addictive" Lee Clayton
"Cocaine" (II) Eric Clapton   "Listen to Her Heart" Tom Petty & the Heartbreakers
"White Line Fever" Motörhead

1979 "That Smell" Lynyrd Skynyrd
"Mary Mary" Inner Circle
"Mystic Man" Peter Tosh
"Koka Kola" The Clash

1980 "A Little Cocaine" Lee Clayton
"Gaucho" Steely Dan
"Mama Coca" Chris Spedding   "Della and the Dealer" Hoyt Axton
"Cocaine Cowboy" Terry Allen   "Bad Whiskey and Cocaine" Honeyboy Edwards
"Frosty the Dope Man" Marc Zydiak   "Accuracy" The Cure
"White Lady White Powder" Elton John
"Cocaine Charlie" Atlanta Rhythm Section
"Stay Away from the Cocaine Train" Johnny Paycheck

1981 *"Juncker's Blues"* Michael Bloomfield
"Champagne & Reefer" Muddy Waters
"Come Fly with Me" Abi Ofarim
"Lines" Grace Slick
"Snowman" Abi Ofarim   **1982** *"One Step Ahead of the Blues"* J. J. Cale
"I Like" Heathen Dan
1983 *"White Lines"* Grandmaster Flash & Melle Mel
"White Horse" Laid Back
"Cocaine Decisions" Frank Zappa
"In the Arms of Cocaine" Hank Williams Jr.
"Rush Rush" Debbie Harry

1984 *"Smuggler's Blues"* Glenn Frey
1985 *"Are There Any More Real Cowboys?"* Neil Young
"Vice" Grandmaster Melle Mel
"Girl (Cocaine) That's Your Life" Too $hort
"Coke Dealers" Too $hort
1986 *"Cool the Engines"* Boston
"Coco Don't" Don Johnson   **1987** *"My Bag"* Lloyd Cole
"Wild Wild Life" Talking Heads
"Cocaine Sex" Renegade Soundwave
"Sign o' the Times" Prince
1988 *"Your Only Friend"* Phuture
"Running with a Bad Crowd" Savoy Browne
"Everybody Knows" Leonard Cohen
1989 *"Cocaine Eyes"* Neil Young   *"I'm Your Pusher"* Ice T
"Prince of Darkness" Indigo Girls
"Crack City" Tin Machine
"Cocaine Lil" Mekons
"Dr. Feelgood" Mötley Crüe

1990 *"Cocaine Rock"* Country Joe McDonald
"Make Your Own Way" Cinderella
"Blow by Blow" T.S.O.L.
"Candy" T.S.O.L.
"No Coke" Dr. Alban
"Junkers Blues" Willy DeVille
1991 *"Cool Touch"* Leo Sayer
"New Jack Hustler" Ice T
"You Could Be Mine" Guns n' Roses
"In the Dust" 2 Live Crew
"Crack Cocaine" Tommi Stumpff
"Cocaine Go Away" Warren Ceasar & Creole Zydeco Snap

1992 "The Future" Leonard Cohen
"The Winner Loses" Body Count
"Pocket Full of Stones" Underground Kingz
"Cocaine in the Back of the Ride" Underground Kingz
"Miss Cocaine" Pops Staples
"Ron's Got the Cocaine" The Supersuckers
"Eyes of Tomorrow" Cro-Mags
1993 "Dancin' with Lady Cocaine" Dajana Loves Paisly
"Crack in the Egg" GWAR
"Crack Rock Steady" Choking Victim
"Bales of Cocaine" Reverend Horton Heat
"Cocaine Princess" Paul Geremia
"15 Minutes of Fame" Sheep on Drugs

1994 "Nutsymtom" 311
"Loser" Beck
1995 "Twisted World" Sir Douglas Quintet
"Morning Glory" Oasis   "Original Man" Andrew Tosh
"Misdirected Hostility" 311   "Cocaine Annie" Gary B. B. Coleman
"I Get the Coke" Temper Tantrum   "Cocaine Jesus" Sister Machine Gun
"MTV Makes Me Want to Smoke Crack" Beck
1996 "United Minds" Arrested Development
"So Strung Out" C-Block   "Line Up" Elastica
"5 O'Clock" Nonchalant
"Don't Sniff Coke" Pato Banton
"Stay Away (Old White Train)" The Fall
"Weed Not Coke" Baby Wayne
"Nature of the Beast" Clarence Spady
"Suicide Note Pt. 1" Pantera
"High Times" Jamiroquai   **1997** "Ghetto D" Master P
"Devil's Haircut" Beck
"Ten Crack Commandments" Notorious B.I.G.
"China White" Grandmaster Melle Mell
"Simply Everyone's Taking Cocaine" Murray Lachlan Young
"South of the Border" Robbie Williams
1998 "Narcotic" Liquido   "One Minute" The Boyz
"Cocaine Lane" Nicole Renée
"Cocaine Socialism" Pulp
"Crack Attack" Fat Joe
"Hoover Street" Rancid
"She's Your Cocaine" Tori Amos

1999 "*Breakfast in Vegas*" Praga Khan
"*Cocaine Business*" Noreaga
"*Cocaine Cowboys*" W.A.S.P.
"*Lit Up*" Buckcherry

2000 "*No Coke*" Rumble Rokkaz
"*Powder*" Three 6 Mafia
"*Cocaine Rodeo*" Mondo Generator
"*Bananas and Blow*" Ween
"*Commercial for Levi*" Placebo
"*Cocaine and Toupees*" Mindless Self Indulgence
"*I Need Drugs*" Necro
"*Who's Got the Crack?*" The Moldy Peaches

2001 "*Cocaine and Camcorders*" UNKLE
"*Bouncing off the Walls*" Sugarcult
"*Crack City Rockers*" Leftöver Crack

2002 "*Cot Damn*" Clipse
"*Coke'n*" Izzy Stradlin
"*How's My Driving Doug Hastings?*" Less Than Jake

2003 "*I Get Along*" The Libertines
"*Peruvian Cocaine*" Immortal Technique
"*Come Undone*" Robbie Williams
"*Elevator Up*" Fountains of Wayne

2004 "*Lua*" Bright Eyes
"*Crack Cocaine*" Pork Dukes
"*Da Blow*" Lil Jon & the Eastside Boyz

2005 "*This Cocaine Makes Me Feel Like I'm on This Song*" System of a Down
"*This Boy*" Franz Ferdinand
"*One Way Ticket*" The Darkness
"*Cocaine Cowgirl*" Matt Mays + El Torpedo
"*Down in a Rabbit Hole*" Bright Eyes

2006 "*La Belle et la Bete*" Babyshambles feat. Kate Moss
"*Viva La White Girl*" Gym Class Heroes
"*Uncle Jonny*" The Killers
"*Song for Clay (Disappear Here)*" Bloc Party
"*Cake*" Lloyd Banks
"*Cocaina*" Busta Rhymes
"*Kilo*" Ghostface Killah

2007 "*Losing My Way*" Justin Timberlake
"*Hotel Song*" Regina Spektor
"*Cocaine (We're All Going to Hell)*" Strata
"*If the Brakeman Turns My Way*" Bright Eyes

FRIEND NUMBER 19
Michael Alig

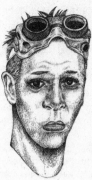

Having just watched Rainer Werner Fassbinder's *The Bitter Tears of Petra von Kant*, the former "it" boy got into a money brawl with Andie "Angel" Melendez, a despised but convenient drug supplier who was living with him at the time. Alig's friend Robert "Freeze" Riggs whacked the dealer in the head with a hammer, then the two poured Draino down Melendez's throat, duct-taped his mouth shut, and put him in the bathroom. Afterward they went shopping. Several days of intense partying later, the stench of Angel's rotting corpse began to overwhelm the apartment. Alig and Riggs consumed ten bags of heroin, sawed off the legs, packed the remains in plastic baggies, and dumped them in the Hudson River. When Alig jokingly bragged about what had happened, it was assumed to be a media stunt until the body later washed up on the Staten Island shore.

Michael Alig (born 1966) was one of New York City's most notorious "club kids" in the 1990s and dominated the city's underground nightlife. Holding court at clubs such as Save the Robots, the Tunnel, and, most famously, the Limelight, the group gave each other names like Jonathan Junkie, Oliver Twisted, Julius Teaser, and Jennytalia and toted their stashes in trademark children's lunchboxes. His on-again, off-again lover was DJ Keoki; one of his friends was James St. James, author of the book *Disco Bloodbath*, which details the glory days of their intoxicated youth. Equipped with considerable charm, a defiant fashion sense, and stunning lack of conscience, Alig clawed his way up to the top of the scene's drug-drenched hierarchy, ignoring collateral damages like the lesbian health-food store manager who he turned into a cocaine dealer and crack addict. The movie *Party Monster* stars Macaulay Culkin as Alig, who was sentenced to ten to twenty years in prison and is up for parole in September 2008.

Alig quit heroin (his last relapse was in prison in 2005) but would not mind taking Xanax again. He is working currently on writing his autobiography, *Aligula*.

DRUGS FROM THE

PHARMACY

Pharmacies carry a variety of different toxins and intoxicants; customers often try to buy them with falsified prescriptions. Favorite compounds include:

▶ OXYCONTIN—The pain reliever contains the opiod oxycodone and induces euphoria. Oxycodone is also available in combination with aspirin (Percodan, Endodan, Roxiprin), paracetamol (Percocet), and ibuprofen (Combunox), but only in very low doses. The dangers surrounding its intravenous use are the same as with heroin and morphine; there is an especially high risk of respiratory depression. On account of its abuse in rural areas of the United States, it's also known as hillbilly heroin.

▶ MODAFINIL—U.S. brand name Provigil; Alertec in Canada. The substance is used in the treatment of narcolepsy and helps people to stay awake, but without the euphoria and exhilaration of drugs such as cocaine and speed. Modafinil is also said to enhance memory and is the U.S. Air Force's new "go pill." Frequent side effects include headaches, nausea, nervousness, and anxiety.

▶ TEMAZEPAM—Known to illegal users as yellow jackets, eggs, green eggs, beans, mazzies, jellies, rugby balls, tams, terms, temazzies, or norries, is a benzodiazepine derivative. It is also prescribed for sleep disorders because of its strong sedative effects. The U.S. Air Force uses it as a "no-go pill" to help its pilots sleep better after a successful mission. Temazepam causes euphoria and is the most highly addictive benzodiazepine. It is often injected to enhance its effects. An overdose can lead to coma. Shaun Ryder claims to have written the entire first album of his band Black Grape on Temazepam. One of the songs is called "Tramazi Parti": *"I got my boots on the back of my head / It's full of jellies in the good old bed."* On the 2007 Happy Mondays comeback album *Uncle Dysfunktional*, Shaun Ryder sings of how, thanks to the "jellybean," he feels like a naked woman sitting in the grass.

▶ METHAQUALONE—Best known under the brand names Quaalude (United States) and Mandrax (Great Britain), methaqualone's euphoric, uninhibiting effects made it extremely popular in the sixties and seventies. "Luding out" became a catch phrase in the rock scene, and Studio 54 owner Steve Rubell was a big fan. Today its recreational use is most widespread in South Africa. Pills are also crushed, mixed with cannabis, and smoked out of a broken-off bottleneck; hence the stripe-shaped burn marks often seen on the hands of Mandrax users. Nicknames: white pipe, buttons, mx, golfsticks, doodies, lizards, loss-of-memory, mind-benders, ewings, genuines, knoppies, magwheels, pressouts, beiruts, wagon wheels, humbles, lula, pupumala, four-strokes, strawberries, flowers, drunken monkey, flamingos, shiny tops, mandies, ludes, Oxford, and Cambridge.

▶RITALIN—Ritalin has an effect similar to amphetamine. It facilitates concentration in hyperactive children and paradoxically it is also calming, since the stimulating effect of the medication reduces the craving for external diversion. Every year, 2.5 million children are prescribed Ritalin in the United States alone. Ritalin is just as addictive as amphetamine and cocaine, and it can lead to paranoid psychosis. The actress Judy Garland took forty Ritalin pills a day near the time of her death.

▶ROHYPNOL—Tranquilizer containing the active ingredient flunitrazepam, which is ten times stronger than the diazepam in Valium. Used by junkies to ease the symptoms of withdrawal and as a post-party drug to come down after taking cocaine, speed, etc. Rohypnol relaxes, paralyzes, and impairs memory function, a combination of effects that has also lead to its use as a "date rape drug."

▶ALPRAZOLAM (XANAX)—Alprazolam is an antianxiety benzodiazepine also used to treat heroin withdrawal (its effects resemble heroin when combined with methadone) and in cases of genital retraction syndrome ("penis panic"), in which a man believes that his genitals are disappearing. The drug was patented in 1969. Xanax soothes the anxiety-ridden mind, allowing it to function more

normally, and is known to bring on a slight euphoria. Combining Xanax with alcohol or other drugs is not recommended and may cause drowsiness. Xanax tends to show the world in a warmer, softer light and is considered only slightly habit-forming. Famous Xanax users have included Stephen King, rapper Lil Wayne, and WWE wrestler Chris Benoit, who murdered his family after having taken the drug.

▶ULTRAM—The active ingredient Tramadol is one of the few opiods not considered a controlled substance in the United States. It works as both a painkiller and mild antidepressant, and can be great for sweet dreams in the right doses. Many junkies consider it too expensive.

▶ZOLOFT—The active ingredient sertraline is an antidepressant, working as a serotonin reuptake inhibitor.

▶PROZAC—Active ingredient is fluoxetine, a mood elevator with no calming or tranquilizing effects.

▶ACTIQ—An extremely potent painkiller and tranquilizer with a mild raspberry flavor, in lozenge form. The active ingredient fentanyl is significantly stronger than morphine. Pain sufferers are sometimes given the drug intravenously or as a bandage. It occasionally circulates as "china white."

▶TRAZODONE NEURAXPHARM —A psychotropic drug with soothing antidepressive effects.

FRIEND NUMBER 20
Tommy Lee

These days the only thing left in his closet seems to be alcohol, but randy Mötley Crüe drummer Tommy Lee (born 1962) also has an eventful drug career behind him. He describes the 1987 Girls, Girls, Girls tour as the *"raddest time in my life, or at least I think it was, because nothing stands out but a blur of insanity."* For a while they had a dealer following the tour bus with a license plate that said "Dealer." Tucked away in their Gulfstream trailer with black leather interior, stewardesses had to put the *"correct drugs"* on each band member's meal tray: *"For Nikki, white wine and zombie dust—a mix of Halcion, a nervous system sedative, and cocaine, a nervous system stimulant which, when consumed, keeps body awake but shuts brain off. For Vince, sleeping pill. For Mick, vodka. For me, cocktail and zombie dust."* He met Pamela Anderson, who he would marry, while on ecstasy and licked her face as an introduction. Today he warns against the use of cocaine and heroin, occasionally reunites with Anderson, and is fond of his "Jägermeister machine," a bar gadget handy for serving the German herbal liquor. Some "Jägermeister" cocktails Lee recommends: redheaded slut; suck, bang, and blow; liquid cocaine; sex with an alligator; instant mess; and little green man from Mars.

JAZZ MUSICIANS
ARRESTED FOR DRUG OFFENSES IN THE FIFTIES AND SIXTIES

RAY CHARLES (marijuana, heroin, and IV drug use paraphernalia)
GERRY MULLIGAN
STAN GETZ
TADD DAMERON
ANITA O'DAY
BILLIE HOLIDAY
ART PEPPER (went to prison a total of six times)
LESTER YOUNG

RED RODNEY
HAMPTON HAWES (sentenced to ten years in prison for selling heroin)
CHET BAKER
THELONIOUS MONK (got a sixty-day prison sentence for heroin found in his car)
MILES DAVIS
ART BLAKEY

PERCY HEATH
PHIL URSO
MILT JACKSON
ELVIN JONES
CHARLIE PERSIP
CURTIS FULLER
PHILLY JOE JONES
NOTE: Despite several house and body searches, heroin addict Charlie Parker was never convicted.

DRUGS IN CONTEMPORARY

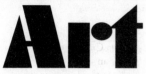

PAWEL ALTHAMER

⦿ *"Remember, you young people. Be careful with drugs. Their effects are very pleasant, but also dangerous, and there is a high price to pay,"* says Althamer, who was filmed on magic mushrooms and peyote and hypnotized for the exhibition *So-called Waves and Other Phenomena of the Mind.*

FRANCIS ALŸS

⦿ In his piece *Narcotourism*, the artist took a different drug every day for eight days in a row, wandered around Copenhagen, and took notes on his sensual impressions; for example: *"Ecstasy. Visual brightness and erotic impulses. My shoes move and I feel the urge to walk out."*

RODNEY GRAHAM

⦿ For the film *Halcion Sleep*, Graham took a tranquilizer and slept in the back seat of his car while being driven around Vancouver. A later work shows him riding a bicycle through the Tiergarten in Berlin on LSD.

CARSTEN HÖLLER

⦿ Oversized fly agaric mushrooms hanging from the ceiling in *Upside-Down Mushroom Room* simulate a perceptual shift; a short film also shows the artist reenacting a bicycle ride by LSD inventor Albert Hofmann.

TERENCE KOH

⦿ The Beijing-born artist also known as Asian Punk Boy titled a 2006 plastic sculpture *Cokehead*: a classic cast bust of Hermes, the god of travel, coated in sugar and diamond dust and crumbling away at the base. Seduction and decay, pretty as a picture. During the performance of *God*, white powder was snorted by the perfomer and his extras.

TAKASHI MURAKAMI

⦿ His colorful fantasy figures and flower patterns were cute enough for Louis Vuitton handbags, and yet the mushroom families in his drawings have heavy-lidded eyes and seem both toxic and intoxicated at the same time.

ROXY PAINE

⦿ For *Drug Ziggurat*, New York artist Roxy Paine stacked drugs in order of his acquaintance with them into a nine-foot tower: from Budweiser cans, to glue, to a crown of heroin needles at the top.

CHARLES RAY

⦿ *"With the rotating table piece, I was just smoking too much marijuana . . . trying to work on a still life piece. I kept trying to do that Russian psychokinetics thing where you mentally bend a fork or move a salt shaker. I was working on that for five months and I figured I was moving them, but I wasn't."* The artist also photographed himself on LSD for the 1990 self-portrait *Yes*.

DASH SNOW

⦿ The New York–based downtown notoriety has specialized in documenting his uninhibited party life with polaroids. One of these pictures shows a young man snorting a substance from the penis of another. Snow's favorite pastime is turning hotel rooms into "hamster nests." With artist friends like Ryan McGinley and Dan Colen, he tears apart forty phone books to cover the floor, gets naked, and takes so many drugs that he ends up feeling like a hamster.

FRED TOMASELLI
○ He began incorporating real pills and drugs such as LSD, ecstasy, and mushrooms into his opulent paintings when friends contracted AIDS in the late eighties:

"Drugs had morphed from agents of enlightenment and pleasure to tools of survival."

HERBERT VOLKMANN
○ *"I always had phases where nothing came out. Be it with addictive substances or without,"* says Volkmann. He paints panels of desolation with cut-in lines of cocaine, encrusted bank notes, and a man with several cigarettes hanging out of every facial orifice.

KLAUS WEBER
○ For the exhibition *Ecstasy* in Los Angeles, the artist built a fountain bubbling with homeopathicly diluted LSD water.

FRIEND NUMBER 21
Johnny Depp

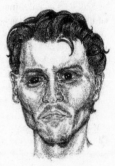

"I think I lived the first thirty-five years of my life in a fog," said the actor. His curriculum vitae is rumored to be similar to his colleague Drew Barrymore's: cigarettes at twelve, lost his virginity at thirteen, alcohol and drugs at fourteen, famous for wrecking hotel rooms in his youth. In an interview, Depp (born 1963) acknowledged the behavior as self-poisoning: *"Anything I could use to feel better. But cocaine is a strange one. I mean, I hated it. You get this synthetic happiness, and then you're just panicking and grinding your teeth. . . ."*

Co-owner of the Los Angeles Viper Room when colleague River Phoenix died at the doorstep of a heroin overdose on October 31, 1993, he later saved Courtney Love's life when she passed out in the club. Johnny Depp's own drug tendency is reflected in his choice of roles: Among others, he played journalist Hunter S. Thompson (*Fear and Loathing in Las Vegas*), cocaine-dealer George Jung (*Blow*), and for the Pirate Jack Sparrow (*Pirates of the Carribean*), he drew inspiration from heroin- and alcohol-bedraggled Keith Richards. Partnered with French singer and actress Vanessa Paradis, Depp asserts that he now only drinks red wine. He changed his tattoo "Winona Forever" (referring to his ex-girlfriend Winona Ryder) to "Wino forever."

GLORIOUS DRUG MOVIES

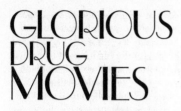

DR. MABUSE, THE GAMBLER (1922)

◉ The famed cocainist Anita Berber doubled the dance parts of cabaret dancer Cara Carozza—will-less instrument of Doctor Mabuse. Two monsters turn their heads toward each other, and she dances ecstatically on their huge noses. Anita Berber said of herself: *"I know exactly what's wrong with me. I'm depraved. I snort cocaine. I already have infected nostrils because of it. Look here."*

THE MAN WITH THE GOLDEN ARM (1955)

◉ The broken, paper cut-out arm on the film poster is a masterpiece by graphic designer Saul Bass. Frank Sinatra plays Frankie Machine, an ex-junkie whose heroin addiction catches up with him again after his release from prison. Frankie wants to be a big band drummer, but his wife, Zosh (Eleanor Parker), pretends to be wheelchair-bound, trying to manipulate him into taking up his old job as a cards dealer. His drug dealer is an elegant devil that injects him with heroin, drives a hard bargain, and in one noteworthy scene explains to Frankie how the only way to kick the habit is to take enough drugs. Sinatra is a skinny little guy in this movie, a prematurely aged babyface with eyes and bottom lip hardened with greed. His portrayal of addiction and withdrawal could be called classic (sweating, cramps, etc.). This was the first Hollywood movie about hard drugs; it brought Sinatra his second Oscar nomination.

ARABESQUE (1966)

◉ Gregory Peck stars as the Egyptologist David Pollock in this somewhat convoluted but very glamorous conspiracy thriller. Pollock is hired to decode an ancient inscription that is of interest to various parties. He is injected with a truth serum in the back of a van, after which he babbles only nonsense and gets tossed out of the vehicle as a result. Pollock totters across the highway, first mistakes an oncoming vehicle for animals of the African plains and then for bulls, inspiring him to assume a torero pose to the swinging sound of composer Henry Mancini. His perception is bleary, doubled, and off-color, but he is fearless nonetheless. He causes a giant rear-end collision, snaps up a bike, and rides against traffic all the way home, where he awakens the next day with a heavy hangover.

THE TRIP (1967)

◉ *"You are about to be involved in a most unusual motion picture experience. It deals fictionally with the hallucinogenic drug LSD. Today the extensive use in black market production of this and other such 'mind-bending chemicals' is of great concern to medical and civil authorities. The illegal manufacture and distribution of these drugs is dangerous and can have fatal consequences."* The grouchy warning at the beginning of this movie, surely not written by screenwriter Jack Nicholson, is somewhat less ambivalent than the original tagline: "A Lovely Sort of Death." Director Roger Corman shows the attractive television commercial director's (Peter Fonda) first experience with LSD in dazzling Technicolor, with beautiful women, old-fashioned visual tricks, and blurred sex, but also anxiety dreams with black knights and ritual murders. A thin, though surprisingly elegant film, despite the closing shot of Fonda's face shattering and swirling around like soup in a bowl.

PSYCH-OUT (1968)

◎ *"Reality . . . reality is a dangerous place"* they say after one flower guy tried to steal the other's girl with an STP drink. Jack Nicholson was of course miscast as "Stoney" the hippie. He can do a lot, but depicting laid-back gentleness is not his strong suit, his stomach was too fat even in 1968, and the ponytail only emphasized his receding hairline. Consistent styling, however, more than makes up for the dullish story revolving around a psychedelic blues rock band and a deaf girl. That and the heavy drug use. Warren, for instance, never comes down from his trip after a night of partying in glittery pearl necklaces with his roommates. He starts to think his friends are zombies and has an urge to amputate their hands with a circular saw. Refreshingly primitive animation technology and a pleasant soundtrack, featuring "Rainy Day Mushroom Pillow" by the Strawberry Alarm Clock.

I LOVE YOU, ALICE B. TOKLAS (1968)

◎ In this comedy starring Peter Sellers, usually rather low-key director Hy Averback goes to show how late-sixties counterculture and the American bourgeoisie can be parodied at the same time. Sellers plays Harold Fine, a Los Angeles lawyer who falls in love with a hippie girl named Nancy and is inspired to leave his respectable life behind. When his unsuspecting parents drop by for a visit, he accidentally serves them pot brownies. Increasingly ecstatic eating noises and rapid brownie snacking are shown with reckless goofiness. The scene is a harmless variation of the then-widespread hope of securing world peace by slipping LSD into the president's tea.

EASY RIDER (1969)

◎ Two bikers, played by Peter Fonda and Dennis Hopper, take a cross-country road trip to New Orleans for Mardi Gras. In the evening they sit around the campfire, smoke pot, and talk about UFOs and true freedom. Jack Nicholson also makes a brief appearance, but is soon killed off by hillbillies. Fonda and Hopper survive the attack and pay their respects to the dead by visiting one of their friend's warmly recommended bordellos. But rather than sleep with the two selected prostitutes, they take them to a cemetery and drop LSD instead. The subsequent "trip" is represented by a weirdly edited sequence; the soundtrack alternates between abrupt shrieks and a squeaky female voice reciting the Lord's Prayer. Fonda begs for forgiveness. Hopper and Fonda are later shot by two truckers on the open road.

EL TOPO—THE MOLE (1970)

◎ A nameless hero rides through the desert with a seven-year-old boy wearing nothing but a hat. After a few shootouts, he trades the kid in for a woman who insists on his shooting the best four marksmen in the desert before she gives herself over to him. He manages to do this with a few dirty tricks—the last sharpshooter even shoots himself— but then the woman leaves him for a lesbian. A band of dwarfs and deformed people kidnap him and take him to their cave shelter where they live in exile. When he re-awakens many years later, he eats a bug, kisses an old dwarf woman, and writhes around on the floor. The little people name him their leader in a revolt against their oppressors in the overground city, and a group of old women can be seen raping a black slave. They play Russian roulette in the church. When the dwarfs finally make it into the city, all of them are shot. Only the hero manages to shoot back, forcing the entire population to flee. After that he sets himself on fire. Meanwhile a dwarf has given birth to their mutual child. The Chilean director, Alejandro Jodorowsky, who also invented psycho-magic therapy, said, *"The audiences who go to the movies, must be assassinated, killed, destroyed, and they must leave the theater as new people"* and, *"I ask of cinema what most North Americans ask of psychedelic drugs."*

PERFORMANCE (1970)

◎ *"You'll look funny when you're fifty,"* says the gangster Chas (James Fox) to Mick Jagger as Turner, a washed-up rock star. Turner lives with a two-hundred-year-old Oriental rug and a stuffed polar bear and likes to indulge in occasional group sex. Bragging about how much he hates music, he keeps a microphone and body-hugging hippie stage costume handy just in case. The film by Nicolas Roeg and Donald Cammell flopped with audiences in 1970 but enjoys a certain acclaim today; besides the relatively generous number of sex scenes, drugs and their consequences abound throughout the movie. Anita Pallenberg nibbles a raw mushroom and smokes a joint with Jagger, who is often seen sniffing and fidgeting with his nose. Later they share a fly agaric and put a wig on Chas, and Anita wants to have experimental sex with him to help him get in touch with his feminine side.

SUPERFLY (1972)

◎ *"Look, I know it's a rotten game, but it's the only one The Man left us to play,"* Eddie says to his colleague Youngblood Priest (Ron O'Neal), the not unlikable, small-time pusher who dreams of getting out of the business after his next big deal. It's hard not to think about how many times Quentin Tarantino must have watched this film over and over again, studying up to steal everything there is to know about soundtrack, offhandedness, and style. The latest it becomes clear is when Priest—a woman with a nice-looking bottom lying next to him in bed, African carvings behind them—uses his little coke spoon necklace to take a couple of lines before getting up. This is where black "gangsta" worship began. *"You're gunna give all this up? Eight Track Stereo, color T.V. in every room, and can snort a half a piece of dope every day? That's the American Dream, nigga!"* or so it goes. And actually there's nothing left to say.

<u>CHRISTIANE F.—WE CHILDREN FROM BAHNHOF ZOO</u> (1981)

◎ German director Uli Edel's junkie and baby prostitute confession, *We Children from Bahnhof Zoo*, is the first and only disco movie in which nobody ever dances. When thirteen-year-old Christiane, played by Nadja Brunckhorst, ventures out of her West Berlin housing project to visit Sound, "Europe's most modern discotheque," her way leads straight to the bathroom. Needles are inserted into arms, legs, and once in the neck, and Christiane's boyfriend Detlef looks as adorably shy and affectionate as only Hector Muelas ever could.

<u>GOODFELLAS</u> (1990)

◎ After serving a four-year prison term, gangster boss Paul Cicero (Paul Sorvino) takes underling Henry Hill (Ray Liotta) aside and gives him a very stern warning about drug dealing. Next scene: cocaine galore. Henry's promotion from errand boy to mobster and subsequent end in the Witness Protection Program are based on an authentic story. Martin Scorsese, at the apex of his ability, fuses it into first an epic, then an increasingly frenzied family saga. Near the end of the film you start to wonder if the crew was on cocaine the whole time, with the possible exception of cameraman Michael Ballhaus, whose steadicam shot through the Copacabana nightclub is a nostalgia-inducing example of nondigital wizardry. The occasional freeze frames are just as effective as the druggy soundtrack (Rolling Stones, Devo) and Ray Liotta's feline good looks, bloated from the cocaine and stiffened in a paranoid mask. *"As far back as I can remember, I always wanted to be a gangster,"* he says in the beginning. At the end junkie Sid Vicious bellows "My Way," mocking the mafia "family values" embodied by the mobster-friendly Frank Sinatra.

OTHER NAMES
FOR A

JOINT

J
Jay
Jive Stick
Giggly Stick
Spliff
Blunt (as a cigar)
Bifta
Doobie
Doob
Dutchie
Small Fatty
Fatty Bom Batty
Flaxman Special
Zoot
Left-handed
Cigarette
L
Holy Roller
Magic Bus
Mr. Boom Bizzle
Cat Tail
Pinner
Rope
Reefer
Reef
Porro
G Nigga Roint

ROMEO AND JULIET (1996)

◎ Romeo Montague (Leonardo DiCaprio) and his gang want to go to the annual ball hosted by his family's sworn archenemies the Capulets. His best friend Mercutio makes a sinister speech about love in the ruins of a Verona Beach theater, after which he offers the romantic Romeo a red-heart-printed ecstasy pill on the tip of his pointer finger. The effect is quick to kick in: Everything he sees on the convertible ride to the party is in slow motion, images smear, the party becomes ecstatic (Mercutio as disco diva), bacchanalian (Fulgencio Capulet as a drunken Roman), and threatening (Tybalt as a roaring lion). Romeo holds his head under the faucet in the men's room to cool off. Coming down from his high, he glances through an aquarium of exotic fish and catches sight of Juliet, the love of his still-short life. Even Friar Laurence is a friend of intoxicants; he slices ripe poppy pods while teaching schoolchildren in his greenhouse.

BOOGIE NIGHTS (1997)

◎ The lines of cocaine filmed from beneath a glass table are nice to look at, but things get a lot more interesting when faded porno star Dirk Diggler (Mark Wahlberg) tries to outfox a high-caliber cocaine buyer with his friends. The three are kept sitting by a bodyguard on the sofa while the customer freebases and waves a weapon around at the same time. The shootout that follows is accompanied by Nena's peace anthem "99 Luftballons." Director Paul Thomas Anderson's colorful farce illustrates how the sex industry lost the illusion of a fuller, freer, maybe even artistic life for its actors. And it shows the bitter aftertaste of the good mood drug cocaine.

GO (1999)

◎ Charming, if contrived, episodic film by Doug Liman about a Christmastime drug deal. Noteworthy for one touching scene, in which a young man on ecstasy stands at a grocery store cash register and falls in love with the sound of the electronic scanner. He swipes the products over the device again and again, composing a little MDMA song.

LITTLE MISS SUNSHINE (2006)

◎ The average offbeat American family piles into a VW bus after chubby daughter Olive is invited to a beauty pageant in another state. Perched in the back of the bus behind Olive's suicidal uncle (a renowned Proust scholar), silent brother, and stressed-out mom is her show-stealing grandpa: a heroin-sniffing hell-raiser who advises his teenage grandson to sleep with as many girls as possible, teaches his young granddaughter freaky stage moves, and has a healthy appetite for raunchy porn. Despite a cautionary word to the young about recreational drugs: *"Don't do that stuff. When you're young, you're crazy to do that shit,"* he proudly champions the right among senior citizens, saying that the old are *"crazy not to do it."* Casually toting his stash in a stylish black fanny pack, his eventual death by overdose only underscores a strong lust-for-life character. A fine example of illicit drug use among the elderly; Alan Arkin received an Academy Award for the role.

JOAN VOLLMER ADAMS, 1924–1951
* It all started in her apartment at
419 West 115th Street, New York;
she was later shot by husband
William S. Burroughs
* Speed
* Lived with: Parker, Burroughs,
Ginsberg, Kerouac
* Married to: Burroughs
* Got introduced to speed by: Kerouac

JACK KEROUAC, 1922–1969
(*On the Road*)
* First: Alcohol, speed, marijuana;
later: morphine, heroin,
mescaline, peyote, opium
* Lived with: Adams, Parker,
Burroughs, Ginsberg
* Married to: Parker
* Traveled with: Cassady

EDIE PARKER, 1922–1993,
writer, muse (*You'll Be Okay*)
* Roommate to Joan Vollmer Adams
* First wife of Jack Kerouac
* In his novel *The Town and the City*,
represented as Judie Smith
* Lived with: Adams, Kerouac,
Ginsberg, Burroughs
* Married to: Kerouac

A SUBSTANTIAL HISTORY OF THE

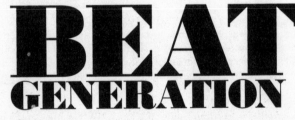

BEAT GENERATION

"*The three biggest threats to America are the Communists, the beatniks, and the egg-heads,*" J. Edgar Hoover said at an FBI convention in 1961. In the early fifties, a handful of American writers, dropouts, and junkies (all at once, though not necessarily in that order) challenged the rules of literature and forever changed the cultural perception of drug users. Their works *On the Road*, *Howl and Other Poems*, and *Naked Lunch* became an indispensable part of subversive young counterculture. No wonder the main members of the beat generation loved and killed, used and abused each other: When hustler and drug expert Herbert Huncke gave William S. Burroughs—who came to his apartment "*dressed like the president of a bank*"—his first shot of morphine, the writer said, "*Well, now, that's very interesting.*"

NEAL CASSADY, 1926–1968,
car thief, muse
❋ Alcohol, peyote, speed,
marijuana, LSD
❋ Traveled cross-country with
Kerouac (*On the Road* characters
Dean Moriarty and Cody Pomeray are
based on him). Moved to San
Francisco in 1952 with his wife,
Carolyn Robinson, grew cannabis
in the North Bay area, and helmed
Ken Kesey's Merry Prankster bus.
❋ Traveled with: Kerouac
❋ Slept with: Ginsberg
❋ Inspired: Ginsberg, Kerouac,
Burroughs

WILLIAM S. BURROUGHS, 1914–1997
(*Junky, Naked Lunch*)
❋ Morphine, heroin, marijuana, alcohol,
yagé, marijuana, oxycodone, chloral
hydrate, firearms
❋ Taught Kerouac how to shoot
morphine and heroin
❋ Lived with: Adams, Ginsberg, Kerouac
❋ Loved: Ginsberg
❋ Married to: Adams (shot her dead)

ALLEN GINSBERG, 1926–1997
(*Howl and Other Poems*)
❋ Morphine, opium, codeine, cocaine,
speed, marijuana, peyote, mescaline,
ether, LSD, ayahuasca
❋ Lived with: Adams, Kerouac,
Burroughs
❋ Loved: Cassady

HERBERT HUNCKE, 1915–1996,
junkie, muse
❋ Speed, marijuana, heroin
❋ Gave Burroughs his first joint
❋ Coined the term *beat*
❋ Became Elmo Hassel in *On the
Road* and Herman in *Junkie*
❋ Shot up with: Burroughs

LAWRENCE FERLINGHETTI,
poet, founder of the
City Lights Bookstore
❋ Single-handedly turned poetry into
a relevant art form again
❋ Defender in lawsuits surrounding
Ginsberg, whose poems were considered
obscene and drug-glorifying
(both true, of course)
❋ Published: Kerouac (*On the Road*),
Ginsberg (*Howl and Other Poems*)

ULTRA VIOLET'S DEATH LIST

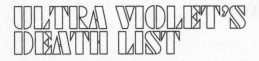

The French artist Isabelle Collin Dufresne, called Ultra Violet, was one of pop art artist Andy Warhol's muses. At the end of her book *Famous for 15 Minutes*, about her time in Warhol's New York Factory, she writes about several companions who died of drug overdoses. Dufresne, who was exorcized as a child, also has dealt with drug dependency and was once declared clinically dead. She currently lives and works as an artist in the south of France and in New York City.

EDIE SEDGWICK

🦇 *"There is no need to say any more about poor, doomed Edie,"* Dufresne writes. Everyone knows she died of a barbiturate overdose.

ERIC EMERSON

🦇 The "pretty, psychedelic playboy" was found dead next to his bicycle. Ultra Violet speculates he died of a heroin overdose.

ROBERT SCULL

🦇 Was one of the most important pop art collectors for a time. Died of diabetes complicated by drug abuse, including cocaine, LSD, Quaaludes, hashish, and opium.

INGRID SUPERSTAR

🦇 Actually, her name was Ingrid von Scheven. After the Factory she started dealing, dabbled in prostitution, and was judged mentally disabled. She walked out of her house on December 7, 1986, leaving her fur coat hanging in the closet and her false teeth in the sink, and disappeared without a trace.

TRUMAN CAPOTE

🦇 According to Dufresne, he died of alcohol, drugs, and *"bodily disintegration."*

TIGER MORSE

🦇 Designed fashions for the Factory and considered herself living proof that speed does not kill. She died of an overdose.

MICKEY RUSKIN

🦇 The art collector and cocainist died of a heart attack.

TAXI

🦇 An early Warhol muse. *"Drugs took her before she could prove her stardom."*

TOM BAKER

🦇 Ultra Violet's partner in the film *I, a Man* died from a speedball (cocaine and heroin) overdose. Not to be confused with the British actor of the same name who starred in the Pasolini film *Canterbury Tales*.

SANDY MARSH

🦇 A close friend of Edie Sedgwick, Marsh jumped from her twenty-eighth-story apartment in 1987 after twenty years of drug consumption. *"Not one, not her husband, her children, her maid, her cook, her nanny could help her find happiness."*

UNCONVENTIONAL WAYS TO TAKE DRUGS

LSD IN THE EYE
✷ Insert the acid directly behind the lower eyelid. The LSD takes effect in a matter of minutes.

SNORTING ECSTASY
✷ Burns something fierce, kicks in faster.

PLUGGING
✷ Administer crystal meth rectally. Also known as: keistering, booty bump, butt rocket.

COCAINE IN A SICK TOOTH
✷ Gottfried Benn (German doctor and poet) recommends "a saturated temporary filling in an affected, specially prepared tooth."

COCAINE ON THE PENIS HEAD/
IN THE VAGINA
✷ These areas absorb the powder like any other mucous membrane. Added factors include the numbing (local anesthetic) effect of cocaine, which on the one hand hinders premature ejaculation, but on the other can lead to mindless boinking ("White Rabbit").

ANAL HASHISH
✷ Insert the hash and coconut oil like a suppository into the hindquarters. Grease liquifies at 86 degrees Fahrenheit; the mucous membranes in the lower intestinal tract can absorb the drug. A bit cumbersome, perhaps.

ECSTASY PUNCH
✷ A Berlin party favorite. Difficult to dose, not unquestionable on account of the alcohol.

OPIUM THROUGH THE SKIN
✷ Apply a vesicating bandage. This will soften the skin and increase blood circulation. Then administer opium.

ILLNESSES AND CONDITIONS CAUSED BY UNCLEAN OR CLOTTED INJECTIONS

★ Abscesses ★ Hemorrhoids ★ Meningitis ★ Cerebritis ★
★ Cerebral mucormycosis ★ Endocarditis ★
★ Cardiac arrest ★ Endophthalmitis ★ Blindness ★
★ Cellulitis ★ Tetanus ★ Gonorrhea ★ HIV ★
★ Syphilis ★ Tuberculosis ★ Hepatitis A, B, C, and D ★

FIVE TEXT EXCERPTS FROM
ARTHUR CONAN DOYLE PROVING THAT

SHERLOCK HOLMES

WAS A COKEHEAD

"THE SIGN OF FOUR"

"Sherlock Holmes took his bottle from the corner of the mantel-piece, and his hypodermic syringe from its neat morocco case. With his long, white, nervous fingers he adjusted the delicate needle and rolled back his left shirtcuff. For some little time his eyes rested thoughtfully upon the sinewy forearm and wrist, all dotted and scarred with innumerable puncture-marks. Finally, he thrust the sharp point home, pressed down the tiny piston, and sank back into the velvet-lined armchair with a long sigh of satisfaction."

"THE YELLOW FACE"

"Save for the occasional use of cocaine, he had no vices, and he only turned to the drug as a protest against the monotony of existence when cases were scanty and the papers uninteresting."

"THE MAN WITH THE TWISTED LIP"

"In a very short time a decrepit figure had emerged from the opium den, and I was walking down the street with Sherlock Holmes. For two streets he shuffled along with a bent back and an uncertain foot. Then, glancing quickly round, he straightened himself out and burst into a hearty fit of laughter.

"'I suppose, Watson,' said he, 'that you imagine that I have added opium-smoking to cocaine injections, and all the other little weaknesses on which you have favoured me with your medical views.'"

"THE FIVE ORANGE PIPS"

"Sherlock: 'If I remember rightly, you on one occasion, in the early days of our friendship, defined my limits in a very precise fashion.' 'Yes,' I answered, laughing. 'It was a singular document. Philosophy, astronomy, and politics were marked at zero, I remember. Botany variable, geology profound as regards the mud-stains from any region within fifty miles of town, chemistry eccentric, anatomy unsystematic, sensational literature and crime records unique, violin-player, boxer, swordsman, lawyer, and self-poisoner by cocaine and tobacco. Those, I think, were the main points of my analysis.'

"Holmes grinned at the last item. 'Well,' he said, 'I say now, as I said then, that a man should keep his little brain-attic stocked with all the furniture that he is likely to use, and the rest he can put away in the lumber-room of his library, where he can get it if he wants it.'"

"A SCANDAL IN BOHEMIA"

"I had seen little of Holmes lately. My marriage had drifted us away from each other. My own complete happiness, and the home-centred interests which rise up around the man who first finds himself master of his own establishment, were sufficient to absorb all my attention, while Holmes, who loathed every form of society with his whole Bohemian soul, remained in our lodgings in Baker Street, buried among his old books, and alternating from week to week between cocaine and ambition, the drowsiness of the drug, and the fierce energy of his own keen nature."

FRIEND NUMBER 22

George Michael

On the night of Monday, February 27, 2006, the singer was found in London's traffic-ridden Hyde Park Corner in his curiously parked Range Rover slumped behind the wheel. The police had been called by two women who had seen him driving his car and described his behavior as *"bewildered, frightened, confused, and apparently under the influence of drugs."* A test showed that George Michael ("Wake Me Up Before You Go Go") had antidepressants in his blood as well as hashish and the narcotic GHB, otherwise known as liquid ecstasy. Charged with driving under the influence, he said, *"I did something very stupid and am very ashamed of doing it."*

George Michael (born 1963 as Georgios Kyriacos Panayiotou) rose to fame in the 1980s with the pop duo Wham! ("Careless Whisper") and later started a very successful solo career until his dispute and split with record label Sony. The obviously homosexual artist kept his private life shrouded in mystery until undercover police in Los Angeles arrested him for cruising a public restroom.

His drug consumption, however, was a bit more casual: While working on his album *Older*, the singer smoked up to twenty-five joints a day to get over the deaths of life partner Anselmo Feleppa and Michael's mother. According to the *Sun*, the police also found various sex toys, masks, and porn videos in the trunk. These, however, are not classified as narcotics by law. On October 1, 2006, Michael, who reportedly hates his fame, was once again found asleep behind the wheel of his car. When later asked about marijuana in an interview, he said, *"This stuff keeps me sane and happy."*

POPULAR DRUGS IN

FOREIGN CULTURES

KATH—YEMEN, NORTHEAST AFRICA

❖ The kath bush (*Catha edulis*) is a plant from the *Celastraceae* family. Its young leaves have a slightly stimulating effect. The user packs the leaves into little wads in his mouth, then re-wets and sucks them over the course of many hours.

IBOGA—CONGO, GABON

❖ *Tabernanthe iboga*, also known as iboga, eboga, eboka, or obona for short, belongs to the *Apocynaceae*, or dogbane, plant family. Iboga root bark is extremely bitter tasting; usually it is chopped in small pieces and chased with copious amounts of water. Smaller doses are a low-level stimulant and aphrodisiac; the body feels lighter and appears to be floating. Higher doses can trigger visions, usually accompanied by nausea and vomiting. The active agent, ibogaine, breaks down only very slowly, with hallucinations lasting for days on end. Discovery of the plants' mind-altering effects has been attributed to the pygmies.

AYAHUASCA OR YAGÉ—AMAZON RAIN FOREST

❖ *Ayahuasca* is a Quechua Indian word meaning "liana of the soul" or "liana of the dead." It refers primarily to a brew made from the ayahuasca liana (*Banisteriopsis caapi*), which contains MAO-inhibiting harmala alkaloids and the DMT-containing chacruna vine (*Psychotria viridis*). Though the hallucinogen DMT is usually immediately broken down by the stomach, the harmala alkaloids in ayahuasca block the active enzymes. When the DMT buzz has let up for an hour or so, Witoto indians in Colombia drink a sip of whiskey or beer to trigger a second flash. One not-so-exotic version of the magic beverage is also available online: Several kinds of acacia trees also contain DMT and can be taken in combination with harmin plant seeds.

BUFOTENIN—SOUTH AMERICA, CENTRAL AMERICA, TEXAS

❖ Bufotenin (from *Bufo*, Latin for "toad") is a hallucinogenic alkaloid on a tryptamine base, closely related to the human neurotransmitter serotonin. It can be found in various plants, but also in skin secretions from the Colorado River Toad (*Bufo marinus*). A psychedelic initiation drink was once prepared from it in Veracruz, though it can also be licked directly from the toad itself. Consumption is not risk-free; bufotenin is also found together with cardiac poisons such as bufotoxin. The toad's skin is also smoked to avoid toxic compounds.

KAVA KAVA—SOUTH PACIFIC

♣ Kava kava or kava pepper (*Piper methysticum*) belongs to the piperaceae, or pepper, plant family. In lower doses, the root bark induces relaxation and euphoria; higher doses cause somnolence. Traditionally the root is prechewed, spat into a container, filled with water, and imbibed. The brew is nauseatingly bitter tasting and it numbs the tongue and lips. Kava kava at its most potent can be found on the small island of Tanna, part of the country Vanuatu (formerly the New Hebrides). Missionaries forbade its use, though after World War II a mysterious, white-clad apparition by the name of John Frum appeared to the islanders, preaching the naturalness of its consumption. Though kava products received an FDA ban in the United States due to potential liver damage, the ban has since been relaxed after studies proved its safety and effectiveness in relieving symptoms such as anxiety. Kava products are legally available as dietary supplements for depression, anxiety, and sleep disorders.

FLY AGARIC—CONIFER AND BIRCH WOODLANDS OF THE NORTHERN HEMISPHERE

♣ Fly agaric or the fly mushroom (*Amanita muscaria*) has been used by Siberian shamans for centuries. The Germanics called it Wotan's flesh and ate it during Yule celebrations. American researcher Gordon Wasson also believes that Soma, mentioned in the Indian Vedics, is none other than fly agaric. Once ingested, the body converts the mushroom's ibotenic acids into the hallucinogenic substance muscimol, the majority of which is excreted in urine. A common practice among Siberian peoples was to drink the mushroom eater's urine. This recycling procedure can be repeated several times. Drinking urine is considered less dangerous than consuming the mushroom itself, since toxins such as muscarin have already been broken down. If the fly agaric user pees in the snow, the scent is said to attract reindeer. Some see this as the potential origin of the Santa Claus mythology (red-white mushroom, reindeer, the trip as a kind of gift). Drying the fly mushroom reduces its toxic potency and exponentially increases its mind-altering effects.

SALVIA DIVINORUM—MEXICO

♣ Salvia, also known as Diviner's Sage or Sage of the Seers, contains the hallucinogen Salvinorin A. The leaves of the plant are either chewed or dried and smoked. Effects can be felt within thirty seconds of smoking the substance, peak for five to ten minutes, and recede within a half hour. When taken orally, effects can be felt within ten minutes and recede after one to two hours. The indigenous Mazatec people in the Mexican state of Oaxaca take *Salvia divinorum* and psilocybin-containing mushrooms at the change of every season. The plant was also popular in the nineties English techno scene. It is widely available in ethnobotanical shops throughout the United States.

PEYOTE—MEXICO

❦ The small, tuber-shaped, and spineless cactus contains mescaline. Nausea and stomach cramping follow shortly after consumption and before the onset of psychedelic effects, which generally last for six to twelve hours. Peyote consumption continues to be part of traditional Indian ceremonies in Mexico. Near the end of the nineteenth century, ritualistic peyote consumption also became common among North American Indians. When Comanche chief Quanah Parker fell ill and could not be helped by the whites' medicine, he drank peyote tea and became well. Thereupon he attempted to unite all Indian tribes with the power of peyote. He founded the Native American Church and started to preach the "peyote road," which swore off alcohol and violence and demanded marital fidelity. The powerful hallucinogen was even administered to two-year-olds. Caution: False peyote is distinctively different in appearance but has—like dozens of other cacti—the same psychedelic effect.

WAYS TO MAKE THE BITTERNESS OF

PEYOTE MORE PALATABLE

❦ Drink unsweetened grapefruit juice while chewing the fruits. The acid neutralizes the bitterness.

❦ Dry the fruits, grind them in a pepper mill, pack the powder into capsules, and swallow with warm water.

❦ Boil the fruits for several hours and swallow the tea in a few hasty gulps.

❦ Mix the fresh or dried fruit with gelatin to make a kind of Jell-O or swallow whole gelatin crystals by the spoonful. The gelatin coats the tongue, shielding the taste buds from the bitterness.

❦ Refrain from eating food for at least six hours before ingesting it.

❦ Infuse it anally as an enema.

❦ Regardless of the method one chooses, vomiting is encouraged if the need arises. Although the Indians believe that a person who is pure of heart is immune to the bitterness, throwing up is seen as a purging of physical and spiritual ills.

DRUG KINGPINS

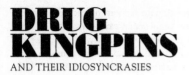

AND THEIR IDIOSYNCRASIES

RAYFUL EDMOND

✱ He was only twenty-four when he was arrested in 1989, but his career as a Washington, D.C., cocaine and crack dealer had been on the fast track for some time. In the late 1980s he controlled as much as 70% of all trade in the region and committed over forty murders with his gang, including that of the Reverend Bynum, who was shot dead while marching in an antidrug demonstration. During the trial it became clear that Edmond spent his money by the bucketful; he dropped $457,619 on designer clothing at the Linea Pitti boutique (the shop owner was later convicted of money laundering). His mother, Constance "Bootsie" Perry, and other family members were also arrested, as accomplices. Edmond is currently in the U.S. Federal Witness Protection Program; his location is unknown.

PABLO ESCOBAR

✱ His criminal career allegedly began the day he started stealing gravestones from cemeteries, grinding off the inscriptions and reselling them in town. At his peak the Colombian Pablo Emilio Escobar Gaviria was listed by *Forbes* magazine as the seventh richest man in the world. Once regarded as the greatest dealer in history, he not only had three Colombian presidential candidates killed, among countless others, but also donated millions to schools and housing projects and purchased flood lights for local soccer fields. His personal menagerie of exotic animals was later opened as a public zoo. Hanging above the entrance to his Los Napoles hacienda was a Piper Cub, the first airplane he sent loaded with cocaine into the United States. In 1991 he turned himself in to Colombian authorities in order to avoid extradition to the United States. *"Terror has triumphed," El Espectador* commented. He was taken to La Catedral prison in his hometown, Envigado, where he lived in the lap of luxury with gourmet cooks, a nightclub, and a bomb shelter.

In his library were videotapes of *The Godfather* and Steve McQueen's *Bullitt*, five Bibles, and books by Graham Greene, Gabriel García Márquez, and the collected works of Stefan Zweig. Escobar began each day with a joint and had a sexual preference for fourteen- and fifteen-year-old girls. He was shot dead by authorities on December 2, 1993—his pursuers trimmed his beard into a Hitler mustache.

CARLOS ENRIQUE LEHDER RIVAS

✱ The half-German son of a Colombian beauty queen spent a large part of his childhood in the United States and had smooth manners and winning good looks. He met George Jung in prison (grand theft auto plus two hundred pounds of marijuana in the trunk), and the two went into business together, organizing cocaine smuggles into the United States. Lehder was insatiably ambitious, succeeded in smuggling huge amounts of Pablo Escobar's cocaine into the United States, and even used his own mother as a courier. He took over the Bahaman island Norman's Cay and turned it into a major smuggling hub, securing it with German bodyguards and Doberman pinschers. Lehder was apprehended in 1987 at a ranch in Rio Negro; just months before, he told a TV journalist that cocaine was the Latin American "atomic bomb" that he wanted to drop on the United States. Federal prosecutor Robert Merkle remarked that Lehder did for drug dealing what Henry Ford did for automobiles. Lehder was sentenced to life in prison plus an additional 135 years, but entered the Witness Protection Program on a deal with President Bush. He has not been heard from since.

GRISELDA BLANCO DE TRUJILLO

✳ Killing off three husbands in a row earned her the nickname Black Widow. An active member of the Colombian Medellín cartel, she smuggled 350-pound cocaine shipments in 1974—a large amount at the time. Her gang the Pistoleros developed an execution-style calling card that was to serve them for decades: Motorcycles surrounded a victim's automobile, shot out the rear window in a rain of machine-gun fire, and instantly disappeared into the traffic.

ROBERT FREYMANN

✳ The Beatles dedicated their song "Dr. Robert" to him. Freymann was a German physician practicing in New York. In the 1960s he boasted of having over a hundred celebrity patients, among them John F. Kennedy; his amphetamine-laced "vitamin shots" were a popular favorite. He lost his license in 1968.

GEORGE JUNG

✳ "Some people were movie stars, and some people were rock stars. I was a pot star," he once said of himself. Starting out in the sixties as a marijuana dealer, he met Colombian Carlos Lehder in prison. The two began importing and distributing more and more of the substance over Jung's Los Angeles connection Richard Barile, with Jung earning an estimated $100 million. Near the end of the seventies Lehder began dealing with Barile directly. Jung was arrested in 1987 but was later released as an informant; in 1994 he was once again arrested in Mexico with 550 pounds of marijuana. Jung is currently serving time in New Jersey and is scheduled for release in 2014. The 2001 film *Blow* is based on his life story.

HOWARD MARKS

✳ "I'd get a religious flash and an asexual orgasm every time," the Welshman said of his first transactions as a dealer. Between 1979 and 1988 he controlled approximately 10% of the international marijuana trade and at his peak used forty-three fake names and eighty-nine telephone connections. Marks completed a degree in physics at Oxford (where he was allegedly acquainted with fellow student Bill Clinton) and worked for a time in the British Secret Service. For a long time he used a passport with the alias Mr. Donald Nice. He opened his own travel agency as both a front and a financial investment, eventually making it one of the ten largest in England, and also planned to sell bottled water from the mountains of Wales in Arabia. His prison-penned memoir *Mr. Nice* became a best-seller; Marks smoked many joints on book tours. In 1997 he stood for election to the U.K. parliament on the single issue of cannabis legalization.

KHUN SA

✱ The Burmese drug lord and former leader of the Shan United Army is also called the Opium King on account of his activity in the so-called Golden Triangle. Born in 1930 as Zhang Qifu, he took the name Khun Sa (Prince Prosperous) when his mother married a prince. Khun Sa organized and fought with his own small army at first for, then against, the Burmese government and later controlled parts of Thailand to secure his own opium trade. In 1989 he was charged with smuggling 1,000 tons of heroin in New York—his suggestion was that the country simply buy out his opium production so he wouldn't have to bring it on the market. Khun Sa currently lives as an investor in Rangoon.

MILTON MEZZROW

✱ The white jazz clarinetist never got his break as a musician, but when he moved from Chicago to New York in 1929, his contacts gave him access to the finest Mexican marijuana in town. Mezzrow claimed to have brought the first joint and the first Louis Armstrong record to Harlem. *Mezzrow* became the new term for a fat, well-rolled joint, and *mezz* was street slang for "real," "serious," or "deliberate." Mezzrow himself developed an opium dependency but reformed after Louis Armstrong offered to make him his manager in 1934. In 1940 he was arrested for dealing marijuana and spent three years in jail. Afterward he moved to Paris, where he died in 1972.

DISTINGUISHED OPIUM AND MORPHINE AUTHORS

◎ Charles Baudelaire
◎ Johannes R. Becher
◎ William S. Burroughs
◎ Lord George Gordon Byron
◎ Lewis Carroll
◎ Jean Cocteau
◎ Samuel Taylor Coleridge
◎ Hans Fallada
◎ Jörg Fauser
◎ Heinrich Heine
◎ E.T.A. Hoffmann
◎ John Keats
◎ Klaus Mann
◎ Novalis
◎ Edgar Allan Poe
◎ Thomas De Quincey
◎ Arthur Rimbaud
◎ Friedrich Wilhelm Joseph von Schelling
◎ Friedrich Schlegel
◎ Mary Shelley
◎ Percy Shelley
◎ Francis Thompson
◎ Paul Verlaine

RONALD MIEHLING

❋ The German son of a policeman smuggled Caribbean cocaine via Amsterdam to Hamburg in the late 1980s; soon he was working directly with Colombian producers and had his own gang of distributors and henchmen. He hid in Colombia while on the run from U.S. narcotics detectives, but eventually couldn't take it anymore and wanted to move back to Germany. Authorities caught up with him in Venezuela in 1995 on his way home. In his heyday he bathed in champagne at the Club Aphrodite ("*You needed 400 bottles, I counted 'em*") and had money brought in plastic bags to his house in Norderstedt, where he lived on welfare.

MANUEL NORIEGA

❋ The militaristic leader of the first so-called narcokleptocracy is currently doing time in a Miami prison for drug trafficking. Ascending to power in a 1983 Panamanian military coup, Noriega was an important longtime ally to both the CIA and the United States, who in turn ignored his Medellín cartel involvement. He was tied to numerous assassination attempts, homicides, and torture. Noriega fled during the United States invasion in 1989 and took refuge in the Vatican embassy. U.S. troops attempted to force him out by playing loud rock music, though this was stopped following complaints from the Vatican. Noriega eventually surrendered.

THE OCHOA BROTHERS

❋ The three brothers, Juan David, Fabio, and Jorge, descended from a horse-breeding family and came to form the powerful Medellín drug cartel in the 1980s. They wanted to populate an island on one of their lakes with lions and tigers. The youngest brother, Fabio, confessed in December 1990, saying that he wanted to put an end to "the nightmare" that had become his life, though he was never extradited to the United States and was released shortly thereafter. To this day the brothers live unmolested on their farm and are active advocates of cocaine legalization. Their telephone hold music is a version of the song "The Entertainer."

BRIAN O'DEA

❋ The native Newfoundlander started out in the province as a small-time drug dealer but soon hit it big as a drug trafficker, smuggling marijuana from Great Britain to Canada and later from Asia into the United States. Newfoundland's richest man in the early 1980s, O'Dea gave up the business in 1986 due to growing pressure from drug authorities, and then became addicted himself. An overdose inspired him to kick the habit, and he became a drug and alcohol treatment counselor, though in 1990 he was sentenced to ten years in prison for his earlier activities. He was released after five years and worked as a venture capitalist in Toronto. In 2001 he posted a large ad in the *National Post*, where he used his drug-dealing past in a sales pitch. He also produced the very successful mystery series *Creepy Canada* and wrote his memoirs.

GILBERTO RODRÍGUEZ OREJUELA

✱ Lead a drug ring that was active around the southern Colombian city Cali. His nickname was El Ajedrecista (The Chess Player), his motto *"We don't kill people, we buy them,"* hence the U.S. DEA's designation as *"the kinder, gentler cartel."* They bought all the taxis in town and had drivers inform them of every newcomer and hacked into the computer networks of airlines, credit card companies, and the American embassy. In 1995 they stabbed approximately a third of Colombia's congressmen, and their profit margin was higher than that of Pepsi. Gilberto and his brother Miguel Rodríguez Orejuela were arrested in 1995 but rereleased soon thereafter. The two were extradited to the United States in 2005.

AUGUSTUS OWSLEY STANLEY III

✱ The grandson of a Kentucky senator was a chemist and operated a Berkeley speed lab from 1963 to 1965. When his equipment was confiscated during a police raid, Owsley moved to Los Angeles and proceeded to produce top-quality LSD. The Owsley Tabs were white at first, then blue, and later printed with various colors and patterns that made it easy to distinguish them from cheap imitations. Some had special names like White Lightning or Purple Haze—a double-strength pill produced in honor of Jimi Hendrix and printed with a picture of an owl. Owsley supplied the Grateful Dead with both money and sound equipment. When gangs attempted to buy the entire California ergot crop, Owsley parachuted into the middle of the Human Be-In Festival at Golden Gate Park in January 1967, and gave away 100,000 trips. Leary called him "God's Secret Agent."

ADULTS USING Cocaine (percent of population)	ADULTS USING Cannabis (percent of population)
GLOBAL AVERAGE: 0.3%	GLOBAL AVERAGE: 3.8%
SINGAPORE: .0002% (2004)	SINGAPORE: .004% (2004)
MACEDONIA: .08% (2005)	BRAZIL: 1% (2001)
JAPAN: .3% (2005)	INDIA: 3.2% (2000)
ISRAEL: .6% (2005)	MOROCCO: 4.2% (2004)
COLOMBIA: .8% (2003)	GERMANY: 6.9% (2003)
GERMANY: 1% (2003)	JAMAICA: 10.7% (2001)
AUSTRALIA: 1.2% (2004)	ITALY: 11.2% (2005)
PANAMA: 1.2%	UNITED STATES: 12.6% (2005)
UNITED STATES: 2.8% (2005)	CYPRUS: 14.1% (2003)
SPAIN: 3%	CANADA: 16.8% (2004)
Estimated figures from the UN 2007 World Drug Report	ZAMBIA: 17.7% (2003)

FRIEND NUMBER 23
Lindsay Lohan

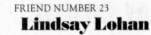

"*It's so weird that I went to rehab,*" the actress said in an interview. "*I always said I would die before I went to rehab.*" In January 2007 she had changed her mind and checked into a clinic for substance abuse treatment. Just four months later, she was in a car accident and police found cocaine in her Mercedes SL-65 convertible. Lohan checked into rehab again.

Lindsay Lohan (born 1986) started her career as a child fashion model and appeared on the soap opera *Another World* at the age of ten. Though she comes from a relatively well-off family, her father, Michael Lohan, also spent time in prison for security fraud. Lohan's parents divorced in 2004, and her mother, a former Wall Street analyst, now manages her daughter's career. At eighteen the actress famously starred in *Mean Girls*, a middlebrow high school comedy, in which Lohan plays an innocent "new kid" from Africa who only too soon adapts to the psychologically vicious world of twenty-first-century American teenage life.

The starlet's mother explained that Lohan gets bored when she's not working, though apparently work does nothing to keep her from looking for distractions. While shooting the movie *Georgia Rule* in New York, the actress was notorious for appearing late to the set or not at all. One of the producers expressed his frustration in a well-publicized open letter: "*We are well aware that your ongoing all night heavy partying is the real reason for your so-called 'exhaustion.'*"

Lohan is closely associated with a handful of American "celebutantes" famous for deviant and drug-consuming behavior. Britney Spears's struggles with underwear, weight, and booze, Nicole Richie's dramatic weight loss, and Paris Hilton's notorious debauches have been important parts of the stories they are selling, overshadowing if not replacing their creative efforts. Lohan is the bad girl everybody wants to be once in a while— but then again, maybe not. In summer 2007, a friend filmed her doing cocaine at Teddy's nightclub in Hollywood's Roosevelt Hotel. After a few lines the actress could be heard saying, "*Tomorrow I go to New York to fuck Jude Law.*" Her friend says that she only published the video to help Lohan come to her senses. After Lohan was arrested for driving drunk and carrying "a small amount of cocaine" in the car in July, her lawyer said, "*Addiction is a terrible and vicious disease.*"

SELECTED HYMNS TO **ALCOHOL**

Hefner: *"The Hymn for the Alcohol"*
Alan Jackson: *"Pop a Top"*
Frank Sinatra: *"One for My Baby"*
The Queers: *"I Only Drink Bud"*
Snoop Dog: *"Gin & Juice"*
AC/DC: *"Have a Drink on Me"*
Cream: *"Strange Brew"*
John Lee Hooker: *"One Bourbon, One Scotch, One Beer"*
Tom T. Hall: *"I Like Beer"*
The Hillbilly Hellcats: *"I Like Whiskey"*
Reverend Horton Heat: *"Beer"*
Highway 101: *"Whiskey If You Were a Woman"*
Willie Nelson: *"I Gotta Get Drunk"*
George Thorogood: *"I Drink Alone"*
Shelly West: *"Jose Cuervo"*
Fishbone: *"Alcoholic"*
Beck: *"Alcohol"*
The Kinks: *"Alcohol"*
Butthole Surfers: *"Alcohol"*
Toby Keith: *"Nights I Can't Remember, Friends I'll Never Forget"*
Start Trouble: *"Alcohol My Only Friend"*
Richard Thompson: *"God Loves a Drunk"*
Bob Dylan: *"I Shall Be Free"*
Duff McKagan: *"Beautiful Disease"*
NOFX: *"Go to Work Wasted"*

HOW TO FOLD A COCAINE PACKET

Paper selection is the key: not too thick and as smooth as possible. Fold the square piece of paper diagonally, then fold the left and right corners inward with the tips pointing toward each other and insert one flap into the other's crease. The upper edges are pulled downward and tucked inside.

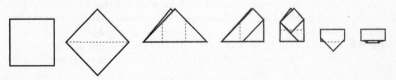

THE BEATLES' DRUG CHRONICLE

1960 An older fellow musician offers the Beatles grass. After smoking they giggle a lot.

1964 On their U.S. tour, the Beatles smoke pot with Bob Dylan at the New Yorker Delmonico Hotel and develop a taste for it.

1965 At home in his pseudo-Tudor estate in Kenwood, John Lennon cozies up with a Quality Street candy tin full of hashish and gets fatter and fatter. The Beatles share a joint in the bathroom at Buckingham Palace before Queen Elizabeth II appoints them Members of the Order of the British Empire.

1966 At work on the *Revolver* recordings, sound engineer Ian Sommerville keeps the clay pipe full of Moroccan hashish. Art dealer Robert Fraser introduces Paul McCartney to cocaine. McCartney assures his colleagues: "Don't worry, I've got it under control."

1967 Paul McCartney finds God on LSD: *"It would mean a whole new world if the politicians would take LSD. There wouldn't be any more war or poverty or famine."* Later he takes LSD with John Lennon, who took hundreds of trips while working on *Sgt. Pepper's Lonely Hearts Club Band,* and both *"saw the bond of their mutual love, and the divergences that would break them apart"* (*Rolling Stone*). Beatles manager Brian Epstein dies of an overdose of sleeping pills and alcohol, a possible suicide. George Harrison trips with the hippies in Golden Gate Park. While he was on LSD, he was given a guitar and tried to fumble his way through "Baby You're a Rich Man." *"It was full of hideous, spotty little teenagers,"* he later said. *"It turned me right off the whole scene."*

1968 High on LSD and heroin, John Lennon comes into Apple Music's London office and declares that he is Jesus. Forty policemen arrest John Lennon and Yoko Ono after hashish was discovered in a raid of Lennon's apartment. Jimi Hendrix had lived in the apartment previously. Lennon maintained that he had gone to great lengths to ensure that the rooms were clean and claims to have been framed.

1972 and **1973** Paul McCartney is twice convicted of marijuana possession and is subsequently denied a Japanese visa several times.

1980 The notoriously thorough Japanese customs find 200 grams of marijuana in McCartney's luggage. McCartney is expelled from the country, and the tour with his band Wings is cancelled. Later the FBI admitted to leading McCartney into a trap. The marijuana had apparently been found at the airport in the United States and Japanese customs was informed.

1990 Ringo Starr quits drinking after going through rehabilitation. For years he drank a bottle of vodka and a bottle of cognac daily, before switching to wine.

FRIEND NUMBER 24
Elton John

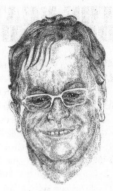

The singer said cocaine was the first drug he took and liked: *"I did not know how to speak to anyone unless I had a nose full of cocaine."* In the long period spent struggling with both a receding hairline and knack for style overkill, the pop star managed to be voted both "worst dressed woman" and "worst dressed man" in the seventies. He also sold over 250 million records and penned the signature hits "Tiny Dancer," "Someone Saved My Life Tonight," and "Your Song."

Elton John (born 1947) took massive amounts of cocaine (up to every four minutes), and was an alcoholic and bulimic. *"Sex on cocaine is great. It's the best aphrodisiac that I've tried. And I've tried a lot,"* John said. He does, however, claim that none of his hits were written while on drugs. In the 1980s, the addict found solace in "Don't Give Up," the Peter Gabriel and Kate Bush duet: *"I listened to that song over and over and cried. They wanted to tell me something and I couldn't hear."* He continues to have cocaine dreams to this day and has said that he can sometimes taste the drug in his throat when he wakes up in the morning.

In 1987 the star was forced to undergo surgery on his vocal cords for a condition that he traced back to excessive use of marijuana. In 1990 he was treated for alcohol and cocaine abuse and received a hair transplant. Since then Elton John has devoted himself to helping other drug-addicted musicians, standing by Robbie Williams and Ryan Adams. When a musician is troubled by drugs, John jokes that they say, *"Let's phone up Uncle Elt."* He still grows sentimental on the rarest of occasions: *"When I'm flying over the Alps I think, 'that's like all the cocaine I sniffed.'"*

His is a classic case of one addiction replacing another: To this day John is known as a shopaholic. In a lawsuit against his management, it was said that he had spent £293,000 on flowers in a twenty-month period. *"I like flowers,"* said John, whose funeral song, "Goodbye England's Rose," became the bestselling single of all time.

THE DEVIL'S WEED:

TOBACCO

There was an epidemic of tobacco consumption in sixteenth-century Europe, particularly during the Thirty Years' War. A tobacco ban followed in several princedoms, punishable with fines, arrest, beatings, forced labor, branding, and exile. Smokers were even hanged in Lüneberg in 1691—as had already been done in China, Russia, and the Ottoman Empire.

When a ship fire on August 7, 1633, catastrophically spread to the city and destroyed 20,000 Constantinople buildings, the Turkish Sultan Murad IV blamed the blaze on smoking, though the fire was actually caused by a firework launched to celebrate the birth of the sultan's son. The regime's utter failure to control the fire caused such a dangerous swelling of rage in the population that Murad saw occasion to issue a royal decree declaring smoking as the cause. Donning a disguise, he would go to places where tobacco was sold, offer a large amount of money, and as soon as he received it, draw his saber and lop off the seller's head. The fortune of every executed person was seized for the benefit of the sultan.

In Persia, the Shah Abbas the Great (1586–1628) ordered the mangling of his smoking subjects' noses and lips. The smoking ban in China was sidestepped by smoking opium instead. Tobacco was legalized again only when the rulers themselves became smokers and realized how much money in taxes smoking could bring in. Arguably the most widespread and devastating drug known to man in the twentieth century, smoking tobacco has encountered many demonizing monarchs and thinkers along the way. Here are some examples:

A custome lothsome to the eye, hatefull to the Nose, harmefull to the braine, dangerous to the Lungs, and in the blacke stinking fume thereof, neerest resembling the horrible Stigian smoke of the pit that is bottomlesse (. . .) O omnipotent power of Tobacco! And if it could by the smoke thereof chace out devils, as the smoke of Tobias fish did (which I am sure could smel no stronglier) it would serve for a precious Relicke, both for the superstitious Priests, and the insolent Puritanes, to cast out devils withall.

—King James I (1566–1625)

They who smoke tobacco can be compared only to men possessed, who are in need of exorcizing. While their throats belch forth the stinking, poisonous fumes, they remain nonetheless thralls to the tobacco fiend to whom they cling with an idolatrous devotion, exalting him as their god above all others, and striving to entice all they meet to imitate their folly. One thing at least it teaches them, the better to endure the reek of hell.

—German writer Johann Michael Moscherosch (1601–1669)

So soon as a ship with tobacco from overseas comes into port—they can scarce wait till the stinking cargo is unloaded—they take the first boat they can find, and off they go to the vessel. Then a box must be opened and a sample of tobacco cut off from the roll, that they may taste the nasty stuff, into which they stick their teeth as greedily as if it were the daintiest of morsels. (. . .) What difference is there between a smoker and a suicide, except that the one takes longer to kill himself than the other? Because of this perpetual smoking, the pure oil of the lamp of life dries up and disappears, and the fair flame of life itself flickers out, and goes out all because of this barbarous habit.

—Jesuit priest Jakob Balde (1604–1668)

No one shall use tobacco because of a bad habit, whereby one wastes time and money and whereby one becomes a burden to others who do not use it, because of a bad odor and spitting. Yea, this evil is becoming so great that instead of getting out the Bible or the hymnbook for mutual edification, the tobacco pipe is brought out for scandal.

—Unknown, seventeenth-century Dutch Mennonite

WHAT **CANNABIS** HELPS AGAINST

- loss of appetite (also with cancer and immune disorders)
- cramps (also with multiple sclerosis, epilepsy, and cerebral palsy)
- allergies (also hay fever)
- internal pain
- diarrhea
- glaucoma
- asthma
- agitation
- aggression
- tension
- withdrawal symptoms
- thrombosis
- depression
- nausea and vomiting
- migraines
- itching
- neurodermitis
- premenstrual syndrome
- insomnia
- infection

ELEVEN EPISODES OF

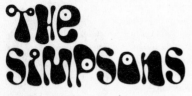

THE SIMPSONS

IN WHICH DRUGS PLAY A ROLE

"BROTHER'S LITTLE HELPER"—Bart is given drugs at school. Now he can concentrate, but he also develops extrasensory abilities and exposes a Major League Baseball conspiracy.

"HOMER LOVES FLANDERS"—Marge Simpson drinks drug-enriched water: She thinks the walls are melting, a turkey comes out of the oven, tells her he thinks he's overdone, and flies out the window.

"HOME SWEET HOMEDIDDLY-DUM-DOODILY"—Marge tests positive for crack and PCP. A second test comes up negative, and she explains that she only needs the love of her children to be high. And maybe a little LSD.

"THE LAST TEMPTATION OF HOMER"—Homer eats bouillon cubes and sees his new colleague Mindy as Botticelli's Venus. Lenny and Carl fly by as putti and jeer: *"What's the matter? Ain't you ever seen a naked chick riding a clam before?"*

"SIDESHOW BOB ROBERTS"—While running for Mayor, Sideshow Bob accuses opponent Quimby of being unable to write and a tax evader, cheating on his wife, smoking hashish, and wasting money. Afterward we see Quimby watering his hashish plants, retorting that he is no illiterate.

"HOMER VS. PATTY AND SELMA"—Barney smokes a cigar without removing the plastic wrapper and sees Sgt. Pepper from the Beatles' album growing out of Homer's back.

"EL VIAJE MISTERIOSO DE NUESTRO JOMER"—Chief Wiggum makes a pot of chili with extra-spicy peppers. Homer eats some of it, his pupils become enormous, and he finds himself in a desert landscape with an Aztec pyramid. An angular coyote speaks to him. Inspired by Carlos Castaneda.

"LAST EXIT TO SPRINGFIELD"—Lisa is anesthetized with laughing gas at the dentist and goes on a Beatles "Yellow Submarine"–inspired hallucinogenic trip.

"BART GETS AN ELEPHANT"—In this episode Bart gets an elephant. His father cleans out the basement, inhales the fumes from the cleaning fluid, and imagines that he's being attacked by their logos.

"HOMER TO THE MAX"—Homer Simpson changes his name to Max Power and meets actor Woody Harrelson, whose pants are made of hemp and look like stitched-together cannabis leaves.

"MISSIONARY: IMPOSSIBLE"—Homer licks toads while working as a missionary in the South Pacific. The effect: twisted eyes and hallucinations.

FRIEND NUMBER 25

Bob Evans

*"Damn it, why can't I be middle of the road? It's either cham-
pagne or sedative time,"* he wrote in his deliciously trashy
memoir, *The Kid Stays in the Picture.* A girlfriend in the
mid-1970s is said to have recommended cocaine for his
constant back troubles. *"What started out as a fuck drug
all but ruined my life of fucking . . . Coming up short
is your cock. Coming up long is dialogue and energy."*
Energy well spent, one could say. Cocaine only boosted Evans's already impressive ego—he hurled his girlfriend's
dildos out of moving cars, showed up at a Jewish friend's costume party
in Nazi uniform, and asked another friend for his newborn son's foreskin.

Robert Evans, born Robert J. Shapera in 1930, moved from being a PR man and
actor to one of Hollywood's most influential producers. He is responsible for cinematic
(and economic) milestones, including *Love Story, The Godfather,* and *Chinatown,*
and counted Jack Nicholson, Henry Kissinger, and Dustin Hoffman among his
close associates.

A German actress he had an affair with was part of a drug-smuggling cartel.
On the way to Malta for the *Popeye* film shoot, he lost a suitcase containing
a few bags of cocaine. To cover his tracks and sneak the luggage unchecked
through customs, Evans told the prime minister that it contained a personal letter from Kissinger. When the suitcase finally arrived (coke intact),
a frightened Evans secretly flew to New York to beg Kissinger for such
a letter, fearing that the Maltese government would cancel the whole
production. He succeeded but lost Kissinger as a friend.

In 1980, Evans was busted in an estimated $19,000 cocaine deal orga-
nized by his brother. As a result, he was sentenced to put his creativity to work for
the War on Drugs and shot a TV show entitled *Get High on Yourself* for half a million
dollars. After one life-threatening alcohol and cocaine incident in May 1989, Evans
checked himself into the Scripps Memorial Hospital to prevent himself from committing suicide. Struggling throughout the nineties, he was never able to match the suc-
cesses of his glory days and battled a heavily sullied reputation. During the production
of *Sliver,* leading lady Sharon Stone said that Evans kept a girlfriend of hers captive for
three and a half years, *"put in a dog collar and chains, drugged up."* Evans defended himself against the allegation, noting that not even his wives had lived with him that long.

In 1998 he married former *Dynasty* actress Catherine Oxenberg. The wedding
video shows him noticeably weakened by medications and a stroke. In the video the
bride hands him a silver bowl with the "Body of Christ": hallucinogenic mushrooms and
peyote buds. Seven days later, the marriage was annulled.

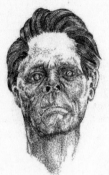

FRIEND NUMBER 26

Brian Wilson

His only regret was having taken LSD. *"It really fouled my mind,"* the Beach Boy said in an interview. Therapist Eugene Landy surely cowrote the majority of the artist's autobiography with a *People* editor just to spin his work with the songwriter in a positive light. For years he attempted to cure Brian Wilson (born 1942)—founding member, creative head, composer, and the Beach Boys' only genius—of his drug, porn, and food addiction. Landy prescribed the often helplessly deranged Wilson psychotropic drugs, a solution that both restored Wilson's ability to work and made him entirely dependent on the doctor.

Wilson's band became the American answer to the Beatles in the 1960s, but it also caused him (with the help of marijuana and LSD) to lose his mind. Business meetings were held in his swimming pool; he played piano in a sandbox. While working on the album *Smile*, studio musicians were made to wear firefighter's helmets and chew vegetables. Paul McCartney, who had dropped by the studios that day, can be heard nibbling a celery stalk in the original takes. The unfinished album was soon shelved and Wilson opened a short-lived health food shop called the Radiant Radish.

In the seventies he consumed large amounts of cocaine, alcohol, and pills and rarely left his bedroom. When he offered an unspecified drug to his daughter Carnie, his wife left with the children.

Wilson, whose *Pet Sounds* is often praised as one of the greatest albums of all time, suffers from bipolar disorder. He only takes mild psycho-pharmaceuticals at present and describes himself as having *"an elevated state of being these days,"* though he has never managed to match his creative peak. *Smile*, which was described in the sixties as a "teenage symphony to God," was released in 2004 after a thirty-seven-year delay.

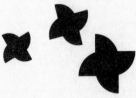

FORMS OF **Alcoholism**

The physiologist Elvin Morton Jellinek (1890–1963) distinguished between five different kinds of alcoholism.

⬤ THE ALPHA TYPE (*Problem Drinker*) drinks to overcome fears, inhibitions, and personal tension. The amount of alcohol consumed depends on how stressful the situation is. Psychological dependence is the primary danger.

⬤ THE BETA TYPE (*Social Drinker*) consumes large amounts of alcohol on social occasions, but remains social and psychologically inconspicuous. Alcohol is a prominent part of his lifestyle, and though he is not necessarily physically addicted, he is in danger of becoming so.

⬤ THE GAMMA TYPE (*Buzz Drinker*) cannot stop drinking, despite having the feeling that he has had enough. He

is in fact alcohol-dependent, despite the ability to maintain longer phases of abstinence.

⬤ THE DELTA TYPE (*Level Drinker*) tries to keep a certain amount of alcohol in his system throughout the day. He is often able to remain socially inconspicuous, as he is seldom noticeably drunk. There is, however, a strong physical dependency, which will eventually result in mental and physical deterioration.

⬤ THE EPSILON TYPE (*Quarterly Drinker*) experiences irregular phases of excessive alcohol consumption and loss of control that sometimes last for days or weeks on end. The urge to drink alcohol is so powerful that even the cheapest bottom-shelf booze or aftershave will do in a pinch. In between benders are sober periods that can last for several months.

WHO USED WHICH
TRUTH SERUM

INQUISITION, EUROPE: NIGHTSHADE + OPIUM
🌿 Nightshade, which contains the sedative scopolamine (example: Angel's Trumpets or Alraune) combined with opium: Resistance is lowered but the person's ability to speak and think are left intact. Opium was also taken by those suspected as a way of protecting themselves against torture.

BANDITS, MEXICO: MEZCAL + OLOLIUQUI
🌿 Ololiuqui is a hallucinogen extracted from the seeds of various morning glories. Dissolved in mezcal, a distilled and fermented agave liquor, it purportedly weakens the will, boosts memory, and sheds light on foul play. This technique was originally developed by

the Indians and adopted by bandits in the twentieth century; they used the drug to force landowners to reveal where their money was hidden.

NAZIS, GERMANY: MEZCALINE
🍃 The Nazis experimented with the synthetically produced hallucinogen at the concentration camps Dachau and Auschwitz.

CIA, UNITED STATES: LSD
🍃 Project MKULTRA (MK is short for Mind Control)—The CIA began testing LSD's effectiveness in producing psychosislike symptoms and as a truth serum. The drug was given to prison inmates and mental hospital patients. Prisoners in Lexington, Kentucky, received morphine or heroin as a reward afterward, so 90% of the participants were eager to volunteer again and again. Relatives of the chemist Frank Olson received $1.25 million in damages after Olson was unwittingly injected with LSD during a test run. He leaped to his death from a tenth-story window several days after the experiment.

SECRET POLICE, WORLDWIDE: SODIUM PENTOTHAL/THIOPENTAL
🍃 A barbiturate and narcotic also used as a lethal injection in U.S. prisons.

BUSINESS DINNERS, CHINA: ALCOHOL
🍃 The Chinese get drunk with business partners as a way of finding out their true motives. The assistant drinks less and reports the next day.

DRUGS TAKEN IN

The Lord of the Rings

TOM BOMBADIL'S DRINK
✖ The jovial Old Forest dweller gives the Hobbits, who have been weakened by attacks from hostile trees, a brew that loosens the tongue but also tastes clear and sweet.

MIRUVOR
✖ The beverage of choice in the elves' valley Rivendell is also a strength tonic. When the Hobbits encounter a thunderstorm in the mountains above Moria, the medicinal drink from Imladris saves their

lives: *"Frodo had hardly swallowed a bit of the warm and fragrant drink before he felt new courage in his heart, and a deep drowsiness departed from his limbs."*

ATHELAS
✖ Also known as Kingsfoil, the substance offers slight protection against injuries inflicted by the nine ring spirits. Aragorn looked for it so that he could ease Frodo's suffering after he got hit by the sword of one of the black knights, and it is later used in the hospital in the

city of Minas Tirith: "... *suddenly the room was filled with a lively freshness, as if the air itself had awoken and was tingling and bubbling with joy. And then he threw the leaves into the bowls of steaming water that had been brought to him, and immediately everyone breathed a sigh of relief.*"

LEMBAS
✘ The Elves of Lothlórien gave the Fellowship of the Ring lembas to give them strength. The substance apparently increases the body's ability to withstand stress by several factors, much like an ultra-strong energy bar or amphetamine.

ENT DRINK
✘ Hobbits Pippin and Merry are given the potion, which has both a sedative and euphoric effect, by one of the treelike Ents they encounter in the enchanted forest of Fangorn: "*I will lie down to prevent the potion from going to my head and making me sleepy.*"

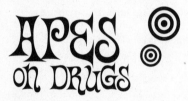

APES ON DRUGS

CANNABIS
◎ Cannabis initially reduces aggression. After three months, the calming effect is lifted and the apes respond by hitting, biting, hunting, and attacking. Lower-order animals that are given cannabis become so aggressive that they climb in the hierarchy.

ALCOHOL
◎ Male apes become very aroused after drinking alcoholic beverages and increase their sexual contacts. In an emergency, they masturbate.

COCAINE
◎ Given round-the-clock access to cocaine, caged apes persist for approximately five days. They then sleep it off, feed, and begin taking the cocaine again. During the high they rock and shiver. Some begin to scratch themselves, bite their hands, and even amputate their own fingers. Given the choice between even a tiny dose of cocaine and sight contact with other apes, they choose the coke. A few apes, even on the brink of starvation, prefer cocaine injections to food.

SPEED
◎ Compulsive repetitive movements replace social interaction. The apes examine every square inch of their cages and bodies, rub themselves heavily, and pull their fur until the skin is almost completely exposed. Ape mothers lose contact with their children and do not respond to cries for help.

MORPHINE
◎ Rhesus apes show reduced aggression amongst themselves. Young baby apes spend more time with their mothers. Spontaneous fights erupt during withdrawal.

Quick Drug Fact Sheet

Cannabis

✱ The hemp intoxicant—available either as a resin (hashish) or in the form of dried buds (marijuana)—contains various so-called cannabinoids. The exact distribution of these and other pastes causes the different kinds of cannabis to vary slightly in their effects (the light, slightly psychedelic Red Lebanese as compared to the heavier, calming Pakistani, for example):

✱ THC (TETRAHYDROCANNABINOL) —Is relaxing, pain relieving, and exhilarating. Slows the pulse rate in tired users, quickens it for alert ones. Intoxicating effects can be felt upward of 20 milligrams THC.

✱ CBD (CANNABIDIOL)—Affects THC by enhancing its sedative effects, slowing and reducing agitation. Hashish contains more CBD than marijuana.

✱ CBN (CANNABINOL)—Product of THC chemical breakdown as a result of exposure to light, oxygen, and heat. Its effects are assumed to be the same as CBD.

✱ THCV/THV (TETRAHYDROCANNABIVARIN) —Faster-acting and more hallucinogenic than THC, though its effects fade more quickly.

Cannabis can be either smoked or digested. It must, however, be heated before eating, which is why it is often mixed

HASHISH:
hash
dope
shit
black
 nougat
nugger
nuggy
piece
peace
chocolate
sticky
sticky icky
faggot
maggie

MARIJUANA:

gangster	t
grass	trees
green	boo
green funk	baby
green penis	airplane
Indian hay	blaze
hydro	lucas
Mary Jane	lamb's bread
Mary	
mj	*Low quality:*
muggles	lows
method	dirt
mint	bunk
murphy	schwag
mota	shit
muta	wag
ganja	oregano
goba	stress
goma	scraps
pot	Lipton's
weed	
weedy	*High*
wacky weed	*quality:*
wacky	chronic
terbacky	chron
ooh-wee	dank
old toby	killer green
Buddha	bud/KGB
funk	kine bud
cheeba	kind bud
banana	kynd bud
ramma	killer
herb	fire
hippie	flame
lettuce	bomb
clone	high grade
(seedless)	purple
diggity	purple haze
kilroy	sizzla
tea	

with cookie or cake dough to mask the strong taste. Cannabis contains just as much tar as tobacco, and the smoke is just as carcinogenic.

HEROIN:
h
lady h
Harry
big harry
big daddy
big bag
brick
gum
chiva
fix
food
hero
horse
aries
antifreeze
Aunt
 Hazel
shore
caca
caballo
junk
smack
thing
material
tar
China
 white
Chinese
rocks
 (crystal-
 line)
brown
 sugar
golden
 brown
negra
nod
noddy
 brown
Bobby
 Brown
boy ballot
black
scag
smack
corgie
cotton
 candy
diesel
dog food
dragon
poppy
pepper
nax
white nurse
white
 horses
wild tiger
sleeper
peg
deathwish
 (espe-
 cially
 strong)
bad bundie
 (inferior)

Heroin

✳ Opium, the milky white "chyle" contained in the poppy plant, contains the active ingredient morphine. Heroin is a product of morphine's reaction to acetic anhydride. The effects of heroin and morphine are identical, only heroin reaches the brain faster.

Heroin was first synthesized in 1874 by British chemist C. R. Alder Wright. It was marketed by the German pharmaceutical company Bayer as a cough and pain reliever and sold under the brand name Heroin (as in heroine) from 1898 to 1958.

Morphine and heroin are dangerous because their calming effects also affect respiration and heartbeat. Heroin is considered more addictive than any other drug. Withdrawal from the substance is an excruciating ordeal associated with extreme physical discomfort.

Cocaine

✳ Chewing coca leaves induces a gentle, uplifting high known to many South American highlanders for centuries. Albert Niemann was the first to isolate coca's active ingredient, cocaine, in 1859; in 1902 Richard Willstätter synthesized it. Cocaine is extracted from coca plant leaves using organic solvents. A quantity of 100 kilograms of coca leaves yields approximately

COCAINE:
coke
cokie
coca cola
co-co puff
c
candy cane
cat's pee
chabbie
champagne
flake
ching
charlie
tony
Pablo
 Escobar
blow
basuco
bah-say
bazooka
Bernice
Bernie
2-5-6
nose candy
stardust
snow
Florida
 snow
heaven dust
gold dust
dust
white
white lady

lady
lady c
white lion
white gold
yuga
yale
yay yay
yo
yeyo
perico
cocorado
shnazzle
skeeter
toot
Lucifer's
  left-nostril
Johnny
Hollywood
hocus pocus
flake
California
  cornflakes
devil's
  dandruff
cover
gooka
happy trails
booger
  sugar
big bloke
bemme
bubble gum
bouncing
  powder
get your
  own
gutter
  glitter
birdie
  powder
angie

1 kilogram of coca paste. A quantity of 20 kilograms of chemicals are needed for every kilogram of coca paste, mainly sulfuric acid, sodium carbonate, and kerosene. Acetone and ether and then salt acid are added to the paste, creating the water-soluble cocaine hydrochloride.

Cocaine is a stimulant that causes euphoria and elevates both pulse and blood pressure. In the worst cases it causes lung collapse or heart failure. The movie *Basic Instinct* was the first to make the sex-cocaine syndrome famous—cardiac death by sex with cocaine. Depression and paranoia often appear after longer periods of use. Cocaine and alcohol combine in the human body to form cocaethylene, which is more potent and longer lasting than cocaine, and therefore even more addictive.

Freebase/ Crack

✳ Cocaine hydrochloride is heated with an added base to produce pure cocaine. The product is not water soluble and therefore not suitable for injection, though it is easier to smoke because it vaporizes at a low temperature and will not burn when heated. Smoked cocaine reaches the brain faster and better than snorted cocaine and the shorter, stronger highs accelerate the addiction. Pure production requires ether, which is highly flammable. To reduce the risk of fire, cocaine is "cooked" with sodium hydrogen carbonate (sodium, baking soda, and Bullrich salt), producing a mixture of table salt and cocaine hydrocarbonate, also known as crack. The

CRACK:
base
base ball
baby t
bad
ice cube
snow
soke
solids
stones
nickels
nickel
  rocks
slab
sleet
Bill Blass
bings
black rock
dime rocks
dimes
bobo
bolo
bones
bone-
  crusher
fries
french
  fries
garbage
  rock
caps
caviar
raw

cloud
crib
dubs doves
egg
forties
gravel
grit
johnson
Kokomo
nugget
paste
piles
pony
glo
press
schoolcraft
scramble
tension
the devil
white
  ghost
white sugar
top gun
troop
yahoo
yale
yimyom
botray
boulya
bumps
bullion

LSD:
trip
acid
a
alice
animal
barrels
battery acid
beast
Big D
black acid
black star
sunshine
black
  sunshine
California
  sunshine
Hawaiian
  sunshine
yellow
  sunshine
haze
purple haze
purple barrels
purple flats
purple hearts
purple ozoline
headlights
heavenly blue
blotter
blotter acid
blotter cube
sid
Sidney
Uncle Sid
royal blues
blue acid
blue barrels
blue chairs
blue cheers
blue heaven

granular "rocks" evaporate at 96 degrees Celsius, causing a crackling sound (hence the name) and thereby release the pure cocaine.

LSD

✻ LSD (Lysergic acid diethylamide) was first developed in 1938 by the Swiss chemist Albert Hofmann. In 1947, the company Sandoz introduced the hallucinogen as Delysid for use by scientists in *"analytical psychotherapy, to elicit release of repressed material and provide mental relaxation, particularly in anxiety states and obsessional neuroses."* LSD is the strongest drug in the world. Effects can be felt after only 25 micrograms, or .000025 grams. Only .01% of the dose actually reaches the brain, making it .0000000025 grams. LSD is either diluted and consumed in drops or the liquid is dropped onto

blue microdot
blue mist
blue moons
blue star
blue vials
white dust
white
  lightning
chief
chocolate
  chips
cid
coffee
brown
  bombers
brown dots
orange barrels
orange cubes
orange haze
orange micro
orange wedges

mellow yellow
strawberries
strawberry
  fields
sugar
sugar cubes
sugar lumps
pink blotters
pink Owsley
pink panther
pink robots
pink wedge
pink witches
cap
conductor
window glass
window pane
grey shields
contact lens
crackers
crystal tea

cubes
cupcakes
d
deeda
domes
dots
double dome
electric
  Kool-Aid
fields
flash
flat blues
ghost
golden dragon
goofy's
ticket
grape parfait
green wedge
zen
zig zag man
hats

hawk
black tabs
instant zen
l
lason sa daga
LBJ
lysergide
one way
Owsley
pane
paper acid
peace
peace tablets
pearly gates
pellets
potato
pure love
recycle
rip
Russian sickles
sacrament
sandoz
smears
snowmen
squirrel
tabs
tail lights
twenty-five
wedding bells
wedges
yellow
yellow dimples
mickey's
microdot
mighty Quinn
mind
  detergent

thick paper and cut into tiny squares, then chewed and swallowed by the user. Feeling the full effects of the trip can take up to two hours. The whole thing should be over and done with after ten hours at the most—otherwise you probably should worry.

MDMA (Ecstasy)

✸ MDMA (Methylenedioxymethamphetamine) was first patented in 1912 by the German chemical company E. Merck, but for a long time no one was really sure what it was good for. Alexander Shulgin was the first to discover its empathy-increasing effects in the late 1960s and recommended it as a helpful aid for psychotherapists. It entered the club scene in Texas in the 1980s. Ecstasy increases dopamine, but mostly the level of serotonin in the brain and has a stimulating, also slightly hallucinogenic effect. Users become more affectionate and have a greater need for physical closeness. Fading effects lead to exhaustion and depression. Serotonin receptors are said to be destroyed even after one-time use. MDMA-related deaths were reported periodically throughout the 1990s.

Amphetamine (Speed)

✸ Amphetamine facilitates adrenaline production but also dopamine to a lesser degree. It was first synthesized in Berlin in 1887 by Romanian chemist Lazar Edeleanu. In 1932, the Smith, Kline & French Company introduced it to the market as a Benzedrine nose inhaler for relief of cold symptoms, hay fever, and asthma. The manufacturers noticed its stimulating effect and launched a new ad campaign in 1935, touting its effectiveness in battling chronic narcolepsy. Amphetamine was used to treat almost forty different types of symptoms (from radiation sickness to opiate addiction and lingering hiccups). Benzedrine was added to the list of poisons when newspapers reported its abuse in 1939, but nevertheless 72 million amphetamine tablets were prescribed to British forces alone in World War II. After the war, amphetamine was sold as a diet aid and given to GIs as a pick-me-up until 1969. In 1971, the annual number of American-made, legally manufactured amphetamine pills climbed to 12 billion. High and frequent amphetamine doses can cause dopamine and serotonin hormone receptors to atrophy and may lead to permanent or long-term depression and lethargy. Only the right-turning amphetamine, dextroamphetamine, reaches the brain. The left-turning version is used in nose sprays.

Methamphetamine (Crystal Meth)

✳ First synthesized in 1893 by Nagayoshi Nagai in Japan, methamphetamine was marketed as Pervitin in Germany and later Methedrine in the United States. Methamphetamine is derived from ephedrine or pseudoephedrine and iodine and raises adrenaline, dopamine, and serotonin levels. For this reason, meth users think of it as having a warmer quality than speed or cocaine. It also more easily penetrates the blood-brain barrier and breaks down slowly. A single dose is effective for up to eight hours. Methamphetamine was used by armies during World War II to increase soldier effectiveness. When the Beatles took "prellies" (Preludin) for their early gigs at the Star Club in Hamburg, their then-manager Peter Brown said that John once "completely lost control," kicked a front-row fan twice in the head, grabbed a steak knife from a nearby table, and hurled it at the youngster.

Methamphetamine is available in powder or crystalline form (crystal meth). A less pure, crumbly form

METH:
amp
alffy
annie
Tina
anything
   going on
20/20
222
bache rock
bache
   knock
bag chasers
baggers
barney dope
Bianca
go
go fast
go pills
blue acid
blue belly
booger
chickin flip-
   pin
chizel
cookies
crank
crystal
chalk
dizzy d
Drano
dummy dust
doodie
eraser dust
glass
ice
gemini
goose egg
hard pep
LA glass
piko
philopon
pure
p
fluff
redneck
   cocaine
Ryan
whiffle dust
white cross
batu
zip
white cross
white house
white
   crunch
trash
laundry
   detergent
nazidope

is called peanut butter crank. A reddish color indicates that it was probably made from red-colored pseudoephedrine tablets, an orange tint points to the use of ephedrine sulphate—some of the ephedrine has turned to sulfur—and brown is oxidized red coloring.

Methamphetamine can be swallowed, snorted, injected, or smoked (like crack)—in a glass pipe or piece of aluminum foil. Teeth grinding, decreased salivation, and malnutrition are common among meth addicts, and these symptoms are hard on their teeth. The term "meth mouth" often applies. Other side effects: weight loss, paranoia, depression, liver failure, cardiac arrest, and heart failure. Excessive meth users are also called tweakers, derived from "all t-weekend long." Methamphetamine is prescribed to treat ADD, ADHD, narcolepsy, and obesity.

2C-B

✹ The phenethylamine was first synthesized by Alexander Shulgin in 1974. The white powder is also often available in tablet form and takes effect after an oral dose of between 5 to 15 milligrams entactogen—like a subdued mixture of LSD and ecstasy. Visual and acoustic hallucinations are less dominant than with LSD, even in higher doses, and can be controlled; the euphorizing element is also less speedy than ecstasy. 2C-B may lead to nausea, dizziness, heart palpitations, and headache. Higher doses of the substance reportedly also cause blackouts. To this day, little is known about the pharmacological and toxicological effects of 2C-B.

As with ecstasy, Shulgin distributed 2C-B among psychiatrists as a therapeutic remedy. After the ecstasy ban in 1985 it was used in the party scene as a legal replacement, only to be banned in 1995 as a Schedule I drug.

Ketamine

✹ Ketamine was discovered as an anesthetic in 1961 by pharmacologist Calvin Stevins and is sold under the brand name Ketanest S. The substance makes it possible to perform larger operations on a patient without interfering with breathing. It also induces the sensation of being detached from one's body and causes hallucinations and feelings of omnipotence. The trancelike state triggered by ketamine is also called k-hole or k-land.

2C-B:
Venus
bees
bromo-
  mescaline
eros
7th heaven
7-Up
Lucky 7
blue mystic
tripstasy
nexus
cloud 9
utopia

KETAMINE:
special k
super k
k
vitamin K
k wire
ketanest
ket
jet
kit-kat
kitty
cat Valium
old man
psychedelic
  heroin
purple
super acid
techno
  smack

DMT

✳ DMT (Dimethyltryptamine) is a powerful hallucinogenic substance found both in plants and (to a small degree) in the human body. It was first synthesized in 1931. The crystalline powder is either smoked in glass pipes or using tin foil. Psychedelic effects can be felt in a matter of seconds and last only between two and five minutes, making it easier for career-oriented users to consume during the work week. Inhaling is often painful due to lingering plant residue (for example, from the tanning agents that color it orange). Unlike LSD or mescaline, DMT also has a numbing effect, and like Parkinson's disease affects the motor cortex. The drug is therefore especially suited to spiritual and out-of-body experiences. Taken orally, DMT is immediately broken down by the body's digestive enzymes unless also combined with MAO inhibitor, as is the case with the South American shamanistic beverage ayahuasca (yagé tea).

PCP (Angel Dust)

✳ PCP (Phencyclidine) was synthesized for the first time in 1926. After its tranquilizing effects were successfully tested on apes, the drug was brought onto the market under the brand name Sernyl (the name was derived from *serenity*) as an anesthesia. Patients given the drug suffered from delirium and psychotic symptoms. In 1965 it was pulled from the market and reintroduced in 1967 as a veterinary anesthesia. PCP can be snorted, swallowed, or smoked. The drug stops all pain, profoundly affects speech and coordination, and causes feelings of invincibility or even greater fear.

SELECTED
Bibliography

ANGER, KENNETH: *Hollywood Babylon: The Legendary Underground Classic of Hollywood's Darkest and Best Kept Secrets*, Bell, 1981

BENJAMIN, WALTER: *On Hashish*, Belknap Press, 2006

BOCKRIS, VICTOR: *Warhol: The Biography*, Da Capo, 1997

BOOTH, MARTIN: *Cannabis: A History*, Picador, 2003

BURROUGHS, WILLIAM S.: *Junkie*, Ace Books, 1953

BURROUGHS, WILLIAM S.: *Naked Lunch*, Grove Atlantic, 2001 (First published in 1959)

BUSHELL, MICHAELA, HELEN RODISS, AND PAUL SIMPSON: *The Rough Guide to Cult Fiction*, Haymarket Customer Publishing, 2005

CASTANEDA, CARLOS: *The Teachings of Don Juan: A Yaqui Way of Knowledge*, Pocket Books, 1974 (First published in 1968)

COLAABAVALA, F. D.: *Hippie Dharma*, Hind Pocket Books, 1974

COLACELLO, BOB: *Holy Terror: Andy Warhol Close Up*, Cooper Square Press, 1999 (First published in 1990)

COOPER, DENNIS: *Frisk*, Grove Press, 1991

CROWLEY, ALEISTER: *Diary of a Drug Fiend*, Weiser Books, 2006 (First published in 1922)

DICK, PHILIP K.: *A Scanner Darkly*, Doubleday, 1977

DICK, PHILIP K.: *The Three Stigmata of Palmer Eldritch*, Doubleday, 1964

DUSEK-GIRDANO, DOROTHY, AND DANIEL A. GIRDANO: *Drugs: A Factual Account*, 3rd Edition, Newbery Award Records/Random House, 1980 (First published in 1972)

EBIN, DAVID: *The Drug Experience: First-Person Accounts of Addicts, Writers, Scientists, and Others*, The Orion Press, 1961

ELLIS, BRET EASTON: *The Rules of Attraction*, Vintage, 1998

EVANS, ROBERT: *The Kid Stays in the Picture*, Hyperion, 1994

FREY, JAMES: *A Million Little Pieces*, Anchor Books, 2004

GAHLINGER, PAUL: *Illegal Drugs: A Complete Guide to Their History, Chemistry, Use, and Abuse*, Plume, 2004 (First published in 2001)

GOTTLIEB, ADAM: *Cannabis Underground Library—Seven Rare Classics*, Ronin Publishing, 2000 (First published in 1980)

HADEN-GUEST, ANTHONY: *The Last Party: Studio 54, Disco, and the Culture of the Night*, William Morrow and Co., 1997

HERER, JACK: *The Emperor Wears No Clothes: The Authoritative Historical Record of Cannabis and the Conspiracy against Marijuana*, Ah Ha Publishing, 1985

HOLLAND, JULIE, ED.: *Ecstasy: The Complete Guide: A Comprehensive Look at the Risks and Benefits of MDMA*, Park Street Press, 2001

JONES, NICK: *Spliffs: A Celebration of Cannabis Culture*, Black Dog & Leventhal Publishers, 2004

JOY, DAN: *Psychedelic Underground Library: Nine Rare Classics*, Ronin Publishing, 1998 (First published in 1970)

KUHN, CYNTHIA, SCOTT SWARTZ-WELDER, AND WILKIE WILSON: *Buzzed: The Straight Facts about the Most Used and Abused Drugs from Alcohol to Ecstasy*, W. W. Norton, 1998

LEARY, TIMOTHY: *The Politics of Ecstasy*, Ronin Publishing, 1998 (First published in 1980)

LENDLER, IAN: *Alcoholica Esoterica: A Collection of Useful and Useless Information as It Relates to the History and Consumption of All Manner of Booze*, Penguin, 2005

MCKENNA, TERENCE: *Food of the Gods: The Search for the Original Tree of Knowledge: A Radical History of Plants, Drugs, and Human Evolution*, Bantam, 1992

MOFFITT, ATHOL, JOHN MALOUF, AND CRAIG THOMPSON: *Drug Precipice: Illicit Drugs, Worsening Problems, Organised Crime, and Fallacies of Legalisation Solutions*, University of New South Wales Press (UNSW Press), 1998

NOCENTI, ANNIE, AND RUTH BALDWIN: *The High Times Reader*, Nation Books, 2004

PINCHBECK, DANIEL: *2012: The Return of Quetzalcoatl*, Jeremy P. Tarcher/Penguin, 2006

PINCHBECK, DANIEL: *Breaking Open the Head*, Broadway Books, 2002

SCHIMMEL, PAUL, AND LISA GABRIELLE MARK, EDS: *Ecstasy: In and About Altered States*, MIT Press, 2005

SCHULTES, RICHARD EVANS, ALBERT HOFMANN, AND CHRISTIAN RÄTSCH: *Plants of the Gods: Their Sacred, Healing, and Hallucinogenic Powers*, Healing Arts Press, 2001

SHULGIN, ALEXANDER, AND ANNE SHULGIN: *Pihkal: A Chemical Love Story*, Transform Press, 2003 (First published in 1991)

SIEGEL, RONALD K.: *Intoxication*, Dutton, 1989

SIEGEL, RONALD K.: *Whispers: The Voices of Paranoia*, Crown Publishers, 1994

SILVERMAN, HAROLD M.: *The Pill Book*, 12th Edition, Bantam Books, 2006 (First published in 1979)

SOLOMON, DAVID, ED.: *LSD: The Consciousness-Expanding Drug*, Putnam, 1964

STREATFEILD, DOMINIC: *Cocain: An Unauthorized Biography*, Picador, 2001

SULLUM, JACOB: *Saying Yes: In Defense of Drug Use*, Jeremy P. Tarcher/Penguin, 2004

TORGOFF, MARTIN: *Can't Find My Way Home: America in the Great Stoned Age, 1945–2000*, Simon and Schuster, 2004

ULTRA VIOLET: *Famous for 15 Minutes: My Years with Andy Warhol*, Backinprint.com, 2004 (First published in 1988)

WOLFE, TOM: *The Electric Kool-Aid Acid Test*, Bantham Books, 1968

Index

Acknowledgments

Bans are not particularly helpful when it comes to better understanding drugs and their effects. In the interest of protecting one's own career, he who researches illegal substances is wise to conceal having taken them himself. We are all the more grateful to everyone who has helped us through the dense thicket of legends, rumors, and smatterings—even if it only meant getting more lost within it.

☺ We would like to thank David Cashion, Emily Haynes, and especially Patrick Nolan.

☺ Thomas Lindemann for research, Amy Patton for research and translation, and Shingo Kuchiki and Brook Banham for the illustrations.

☺ Judith Banham for the trippy design.

☺ Conversation partners, informants, and friends: Tenzing Barshee, Roger Bundschuh, Dr. Pierre-Arnaud Chouvy, Dr. Peter D. A. Cohen, Frauke Finsterwalder, Winni Fleckner, Neal Franc, Mathias Gatza, Barbara Gies, Torston E. Höhle, Rafael Horzon, Heiko Keinath, Prof. Wolf Kemper, Matthias Kind, Olrik Kleiner, Henning Kober, Lucas Koch, Emanuel Kotzian, Christian Kracht, Marcelo Krasilcic, Irina Kromayer, Georg Lauer, David Lieske, Dieter Maul, Eva Munz, Michel Opladen, Dr. Bettina Paul, Mary Louise and Andrew Pearlman, Markus Peichl, Daniel Pinchbeck, Cay-Sophie Rabinowitz, Dr. Christian Rätsch, Christian Rattemeyer, Eran Rothschild, Prof. Dr. Sebastian Scheerer, André Schlechtriem, Alexander Schröder, Yasmine Schröder-Elgarafi, Paul Snowden, Prof. Dr. Fritz Sörgel, Bernhard Stellmacher, Prof. Dr. Rainer Thomasius, Wolfgang Tress, Trikont, Felix Velasco, Katrin Vellrath, Herbert Volkmann, Armin von Milch, Annika von Taube, Thilo Wermke, Theo Wimhöfer, Jan Christoph Wolter, and Gernot Wozak.

☺ Our very special thanks to Antje and Frank.